Positive Spirituality
in Health Care

Nine Practical Approaches to Pursuing
Wholeness for Clinicians, Patients, and
Health Care Organizations

Positive Spirituality in Health Care

Nine Practical Approaches to Pursuing Wholeness for Clinicians, Patients, and Health Care Organizations

Frederic C. Craigie, Jr., PhD

Maine-Dartmouth Family Medicine Residency,
Dartmouth Medical School,
and
Arizona Center for Integrative Medicine,
University of Arizona College of Medicine

MILL CITY PRESS
MINNEAPOLIS, MN

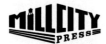

Mill City Press, Inc.
212 3rd Avenue North, Suite 290
Minneapolis, MN 55401
612.455.2294
www.millcitypublishing.com

ISBN - 978-1-936107-47-6
ISBN - 1-936107-47-3
LCCN - 2010920704

Cover Design by Wes Moore
Typeset by James Arneson

Cover art © 2008 Caren Loebel-Fried
www.carenloebelfried.com

Printed in the United States of America

To Heather, Matthew, and Tom Craigie.
The spirit and commitments of your lives inspire me
and make the world a better place.

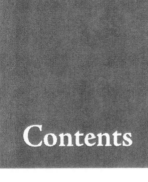

Contents

The Context

- Defining spirituality
- So what, then, *is* spirituality?
- Dimensions of spirituality
- Suffering

- Spirituality is intimately related to health, wholeness, and well-being
- Spirituality mediates choices in health behaviors
- Spirituality often frames the ways that people cope with adversity and pursue the journey toward wellness/wholeness
- Spirituality is important because people want to be known in this way by their caregivers

Nine Practical Approaches to Bringing Positive Spirituality into Health and Wellness Care

Personal: Connections with What Matters to You

Clinical: Connections with What Matters to Your Patients

Organizational: Connecting with the Shared Energy of People Working Together

Index of Strategies

Acknowledgments

Anyone who looks back along a journey that has been worth taking can see a remarkable collection of fellow travelers who have offered encouragement and support. This is certainly the case with me. My closest associates in the work of spirituality and health care in the last several years have been my faculty colleagues at the Arizona Center for Integrative Medicine; Howard Silverman, MD MS, David Rychener, PhD, Victoria Maizes, MD, Tieraona Low Dog, MD, Patricia Lebensohn, MD, Moira Andre and Andrew Weil, MD. Thank you all for your friendship, for the affirmation that spirituality is really central on the path toward healing and wholeness, and for your enlightened conversation about how we invite spirit into the work that we do. I am also particularly grateful to Dr. Maizes for her kind and generous Foreword.

My ideas about spirituality and health care have been greatly enriched over the years by the stories and dialogue from the fellows in Integrative Medicine at the Arizona Center for Integrative Medicine. Among many hundreds of such exchanges, I have included material (with generous permission) from Barbara L. Bakus, DO, Angela Lynn Barnett, MD, Katherine Bayliss, MD, Suzanne Bertollo, MD, MPH, Trevor M. Braden, MD, Christine Bugas, DO, Rosemarie Butterfield, MD, Gary Conrad, MD, Kathalina A. Corpus, MD, Deborah A. Dunn, MD, MPH, Susana Escobar, MD, Paula Renee Fayerman, MD, FCFP, Vani Gandhi, MD, Janet Lewis, MD, Jill Mallory, MD, Mark D. Moon MD, David Moss, MD, Amy Pabst, MD, Robert A. Pendergrast, Jr., MD, MPH, Mary Ellen Sabourin, MD, Christina Louise Stroup, MD, MS, and Joseph Zirneskie, MD.

Among my local colleagues and friends, I am ever grateful to three people in whom I always find wisdom and inspiration in the conversation about spirituality and health; Diane S. Campbell, MD, Elizabeth B. Hart, MD, and Richard F. Hobbs, III, MD, FAAFP, DABMA.

My 1996 sabbatical colleagues at the Seton Cove in Austin, Texas, helped with the formation of my ideas about organizational soul and have remained dear to me over the years: Sr. Mary Rose McPhee, DC, Jan and Ed Berger, Leslie Hay, and Travis Froelich.

The leadership and staff of the community health centers in my exemplary practice research will remain anonymous because of the protocols of doing this kind of research. You are still out there, though, providing great health care to Maine people and caring about one another, and you have my sincere respect.

For miscellaneous permissions and words of feedback and support; Amy Madden, MD, Priscilla Abercrombie, RN, NP, PhD, Larry A. Willms, MD CCFP, Harold G. Koenig, MD, MHSc, Sara Roberts, PA-C, Margaret J. Wheatley, EdD, Christina Puchalski, MD, MS (and the George Washington Institute for Spirituality and Health), Everett L. Worthington, Jr., PhD, Robert D. Enright, PhD, Lynn Underwood, PhD, Gowri Anandarajah, MD, Lee G. Bolman, PhD, Kay Gornick (Prairie Home Productions), Renee Anthuis, AAFP, and Douglas Harper (the Online Etymology Dictionary).

Thanks to my community of writers for their feedback and support. Led by the irrepressible Bill O'Hanlon, MS, they also include Mary Beth Averill, LICSW, Ph.D, Sandy Beadle, Adele V. Bradley, MA, LCMHC, Niel Cameron, Hope W. Hawkins, Ryan Nagy, Lisa Robertson, and Robin Temple.

The late David B. Larson, MD was a generous collaborator on early meta-analytic research on spirituality and health, and helped to form my professional direction and passion in this area. The late Thomas Nevola, MD set in motion some conversations in Central Maine that have evolved into a vital Department of Pastoral Care at the Augusta campus of MaineGeneral Medical Center, and a 23-year annual symposium that bears his name.

The cover image, *Tree of Life*, was graciously provided by the artist, Caren Loebel-Fried. The bird nestled in the tree is a phoenix, the mythical firebird that symbolizes renewal in the traditions of many world cultures. Readers can see more of Caren's stunning work at http://www.carenloebelfried.com/. Hearty thanks to the broadly-

Acknowlegments

talented Matthew Craigie for the portrait on the back cover.

Thanks also to Mark Levine and the staff at Mill City Press. A pleasure to work with.

My wife, Beth, remained patient and cheerful over the winter of 2008-2009 with her husband impersonating a piece of furniture, planted ten feet away from the pellet stove, staring at the laptop. She is also among the wisest, most spiritually grounded, and uplifting people I have ever been blessed to know.

Foreword

Physicians and other health care providers are invited into the most intimate moments of people's lives. Birth, death, sexuality, and loss of bodily and mental functions are revealed in the therapeutic union created between patient and clinician. Within this context, but often missed or ignored, are spiritual questions. Buried just below the surface of most clinical encounters lie questions related to meaning, to faith, and to larger existential matters. "Why did this happen to me?" "I have been a devout Christian (Jew, Muslim, etc.); why would God give me cancer?" "My father was a good man; how could he now be stricken with Alzheimer's, with his dignity lost and all that he valued gone?"

Doctors and nurses have often sidestepped these questions as not part of our domain as health care providers. Indeed, many of these questions are not answerable. Rainer Rilke in his timeless book *Letters to a Young Poet* suggests that we learn to "love the questions themselves." While this may be good advice for the questioner, how does it relate to the health professional? By bearing witness, by acknowledging the unspoken questions, we provide an opportunity to our patients for growth. Challenges of all kinds hone our development as human beings. They can serve as tests that provoke us to express our finest selves.

Parallel to our human potential for physical prowess and intellectual capacity, we have a wellspring of spiritual strength from which to draw. This may be of profound importance not only in times of crisis; it may be the waters that sustain us through our ordinary day to day existence as well. Whether wrestling with pain from osteoarthritis, an addiction to alcohol or drugs, a depression, or even boredom, spiritual resources can help us surface from the depths. Indeed, spiritual answers may serve as our most powerful approach to overcome life's obstacles, offering us direction, hope, meaning, and renewal.

Expressions of profound gratitude may also be of a spiritual nature. "I am so deeply grateful for this healthy baby" is not only a common sentiment among new parents; it is often experienced as a spiritual event. The middle-aged woman challenged by years of diabetes may feel similarly blessed to "see my daughter graduate from college."

Health professionals can certainly refer to others with more training, expertise and even comfort. But they must recognize the subtle hints that are often the only expression of the agonizing questions being asked. Medical educators have suggested sets of questions that can be taught to students and residents so that they take a good spiritual history. While these questions serve to enhance comfort and are a good starting point, they may imply that one can either include or exclude a spiritual history the way one decides on the need for a sexual history or a mental status exam depending on the presenting problem. Like Dr. Craigie, I believe the more appropriate model is an embodiment model of spirituality. Framed this way, we acknowledge the presence of the spiritual domain in whatever is going on.

In this wonderfully researched and written book, Dr. Fred Craigie leads by example, weaving together compelling stories that reveal to us how spirituality impacts health. He reviews decades of research and makes a compelling case for health care providers to delve into this part of their patients' lives. He reminds us, with vivid cases, how these conversations enrich our lives as well as those of our patients. He reminds us that our patients want us to be present, to listen generously and with compassion, and to provide realistic hope. While we may all recognize these attributes of good medicine, he points out that when these elements are present, our patients feel spiritually cared for.

Dr. Craigie then proceeds to teach us nine approaches to bringing spirituality into healthcare. He frames his approaches in three domains: personal, clinical, and organizational. The personal reveals how we can stay connected with a higher purpose, how we can cultivate our own character, and ways to ground ourselves in the context of a healing intention. The clinical covers practical approaches to working with patients. This includes history taking and partnering with patients as they discover and pursue what is meaningful to them. It also includes learning to recognize and support transcendence in others. Finally, Dr. Craigie challenges us to include the organizational level by honoring mission and values, by cultivating a workplace community that attends to the spiritual domains, and by exercising empowering leadership.

I have worked with Dr. Craigie for a decade now. He has taught spirituality and medicine in the Fellowship Program at the Arizona Center for Integrative Medicine since its inception in 2000. He is beloved by the more than 500 fellows who studied with him and found his teaching of supreme value. I am confident that you will have a similar experience.

Ultimately, Dr. Craigie enriches us with his years of experience teaching spirituality to health providers. He gives us a frame to use and language we need to help us be more comfortable and focused in providing spiritual care. He reminds us of the value of simply sitting with another human being and witnessing their journey. And in the end, it is our patients who benefit by feeling seen and acknowledged for who they are and for what is important to them.

Victoria Maizes, MD
Executive Director, Arizona Center for Integrative Medicine
Associate Professor of Medicine, Family Medicine, and Public Health
University of Arizona

September 2009

Introduction

"I know that this is important, but I really can't picture myself doing it."

The warm morning sun, along with fresh-roasted Vera Cruz coffee, took the chill out of the air as we sat together in a small outdoor plaza. A circular fountain muffled the sounds of passing cars; craggy mountains were striking against a blue sky in the distance.

My colleague, a family physician, was speaking about her misgivings about incorporating spirituality in her practice of medicine.

"I see how prominent all of this has become..." she said, "... hundreds of articles, courses in medical schools, protocols for spirituality assessment... but it still seems daunting to have those kinds of conversations with the people I see day in and day out."

"Tell me about a patient you have seen in recent times who has touched you in some way," I asked.

She paused, watching a cactus wren swoop down to grab a wayward muffin fragment.

I saw an elderly man in the office with two of his middle aged children, a son and a daughter. A new patient, the first time I had met any of them. The man had had a stroke a few months before and was alert but had great difficulty communicating. His kids brought him in because he was sick... he really looked under the weather... and they were concerned about whether he was developing pneumonia.

I took care of the medical business... he was sick but didn't have pneumonia... and in this visit that was otherwise pretty matter-of-fact, I thought I saw some real tenderness in the way the son helped his father down from the exam table. I said something like "You folks really look fond of your dad... tell me a little about him."

They immediately brightened, telling me how he had raised them as a single parent after the death of their mother and how he had always insisted on being self-employed so he would have the flexibility of being there for them with school and everything else that kids do. We spoke for a short time about a few more details… the dad had worked in the woods, built a modest home, eventually had a small taxi business and was known in his community as someone who would be generous and patient. The daughter concluded, "We never had very much money, but even when we were hungrier than we would want to be, we always knew we were loved."

Hearing this, the dad broke into a broad smile, too. You could see how much he cherished his children, and I think it really meant something to him to have them tell those things to his doctor. When we left the room, they all heartily shook my hand and the children said how glad they were that I was now his doctor.

"In times like those," she reflected, "I am reminded about what a privilege it is to be able to be a part of people's lives."

"I can see," I suggested, "that you already know something about good spiritual care."

HESITATION ABOUT SPIRITUAL CARE

This story is far from unique. My experience is that the health care clinicians I have known… physicians, nurses, behavioral health specialists, alternative medicine practitioners and many others… are generally aware of the rising tide of interest in spirituality in health care, but often lack a clear sense of what this might mean for them. They warm to the *idea* of spirituality in health care, but are not sure how this idea can find its way into the day to day practice of their professional work. Principally, the hesitation about spiritual care that I hear from health care clinicians takes three forms.

Time

First, some clinicians say that they are held back by *time*. The assumption is that good spiritual care requires extended conversations that take more time than the fast pace of health care allows. "I'm booked every ten to fifteen minutes all day," an internist points out;

"How can I make the time to talk with people about their spiritual lives and struggles without ending up staying late into the evening?"

Of course, time can sometimes be an ally in providing spiritual care. The time that clinicians have to get to know someone in a health care visit, and, more broadly, the time that clinicians have to get to know people in continuity relationships can help with the development of healing relationships and the exploration of spiritual issues.

I would argue, however... and we shall discuss... that clock time does not have a necessary relationship with good spiritual care or with healing. In workshops, I sometimes ask participants to identify events in their lives where someone has touched or influenced them in a meaningful way. The stories I hear typically encompass very little time. An unforeseen reaction of charity when someone knew that they had done wrong. A word of recognition about someone's efforts out of the public eye. A comment pointing to inner resources and inviting someone to let their light shine more brightly.

Medical intuitive Caroline Myss PhD reports a dramatic story that was told to her about a patient who had made his way back from very serious depression.[1] The patient said that his healing journey really began when he had decided to kill himself. He had concluded that life was not worth the pain he was feeling and he had worked out plans to end it all. On his way to his appointed demise, he had to walk a few city blocks and found himself stopping at a crosswalk, along with vehicle traffic going the same way. A woman who was driving the first car in line stopped for him and their eyes met. She smiled. He crossed the street and she drove off, but the warmth of that momentary human contact gave him a glimmer of hope and led him to question his plans. The man later recounted that the woman "brought me back to life with that smile." Dr. Myss' comment is that the woman "channeled grace" to the distraught man. A four-second spiritual intervention!

Skills

The second hesitation I hear from health care clinicians about spiritual care has to do with *skills*. The assumption is that good spiritual care requires theological sophistication and specialized knowledge and training in models of spiritual assessment and intervention. "Chaplains spend years learning these things," a social worker asks; "How can I do justice to people's spiritual issues without that kind of background?"

Of course, spiritual care does involve skills. What do you say to a man with a life-compromising illness who tells you that God has abandoned him and he wishes to die? There may not be a single right response to this situation, but some responses are less good or better than others. Skills and approaches to such situations are learnable; perhaps this is why you have picked up this book.

I would suggest, though... as we shall also discuss... that spiritual care by health care givers is not fundamentally defined by skills and techniques. At its foundation, spiritual care by health care givers is about intention and presence. The word I typically use is "embodiment;" the way in which a healing spirit is embodied in the person and presence of the health care giver. You can have the greatest and most sophisticated spiritual skills possible, but without healing intention and compassionate presence, you are likely not to get very far with the abandoned man with the life-threatening illness.

This foundational role of intention and presence should come as good news to health care givers for two reasons. First, there are encouraging data that these things matter in the process of health and healing. Second, most health care givers have these things in spades. I find very consistently that people choose health care careers because it is important to them to make a difference in the lives of other people. The family doctor who was originally a public health nurse in a rural clinic in Guatemala and wanted to learn medicine to be able to serve people in a more substantial way. The medical assistant who works at an inner city clinic in the neighborhood where she grew up as an expression of giving back to her community. The physical therapist who was deeply impressed and appreciative of the care given him by an older physical therapist... now a mentor... who worked with him after a motorcycle accident.

The "origin stories" of people serving in health care often point to events that have cultivated or nurtured a spirit of caring and a commitment to healing. The system of health care, with its administrative demands and productivity requirements, may sometimes dampen this spirit, but in most clinicians, the spirit remains in at least humble form. Even among physicians who are substantially disillusioned with the medical care system, I often hear comments such as, "I really feel bitter and burned out with the superfluous things in my job, but my saving grace is that when I close the door and I'm there with a patient, I feel some of the same energy and joy in connecting with people that I did when I started out."

I believe that affirming the compassionate values and basic people skills that health care givers bring to their work is essential in the conversation about spirituality in health care. Some of the greatest wisdom comes not from outside, but from within.

This book, then, balances affirmation and skill development. Affirmation of the values and skills that are already there, along with conversation about some specific additional approaches that can enhance the ways that health care givers provide spiritual care.

Fear

The final hesitation I hear from health care clinicians about spiritual care has to do with *fear*. Unlike concerns about time and skills, the hesitation about fear is largely unspoken. Health care givers may express some apprehension or concern that engaging in conversations about spiritual topics will take up inordinate and unavailable amounts of time, but the issue of fear runs deeper than that. I think it has to do with fear of invalidation.

Most of us who have graduate degrees and health care credentials have been able to be professionally successful because we are good at controlling the world around us. A physician can orchestrate a multidimensional workup of a series of medical complaints and mobilize a large cast of characters to carry it out. An acupuncturist knows the subtleties of depths and qualities of pulses, which, to the rest of us, would be completely incomprehensible. A caseworker knows the eligibility criteria for various types of health care and public assistance and can work with systems to help patients take advantage of the resources that are available. All of us can generally put our personal feelings and distractions aside in order to do what we need to do.

We take pride in our abilities to know what we are doing. It is a source of validation that we know what we are doing.

Venturing into the uncertain territory of spiritual care calls this into question. An oncologist recounts,

The patient and his wife came back for the second visit after his cancer diagnosis and he said that he was so angry at God for doing this to him... and he certainly was angry. I really didn't have any idea what I could say that would be helpful... do I tell him that God really didn't cause his cancer? Do I just reflect back to him what he said? I think maybe I'd be pretty angry at God, too. The two of them left just as upset as when they came in, and that's hard to take.

For most of us, this is a painful place to be... having had the experience of not knowing what to do, and fearing that we were therefore unable to help somebody at a point of their suffering and need.

I'm not sure that fear completely goes away, and I would not make the claim that this book will enable readers to pursue spiritual care with complete confidence, comfort and assurance. After all, fear is often a fellow traveler on any journey that is worth taking. My hope, however, is that the affirmation that you already bring a great deal of wisdom to this enterprise, along with our exploring together some additional concrete perspectives and skills, will strengthen and empower you in your own unique approach to spiritual care.

SPIRITED CONNECTIONS

The main body of this book is organized into three sections, representing three interrelated arenas in which we may bring positive spirituality into health and wellness care. They are; our *personal* spirituality as clinicians and human beings, the *clinical* approaches we pursue in supporting the spirituality of patients, and the *organizational* spirituality that is expressed in the culture and values of health care organizations.

The personal arena:
Connecting with what matters to you

If the foundation of spiritual care by health care givers is about intention and presence, then our own spirituality holds utmost importance. The issue is not that we need to follow some prescribed or formal spiritual path, but rather that we need to connect with the things in our lives that matter the most to us.

We will review data suggesting that pursuing our own deepest values and cultivating personally meaningful qualities of character promote wholeness and well-being. Do you value compassion? Be compassionate. Do you value gratitude? Be grateful. Do you feel most alive when you are serving somebody else? Serve. Do you pride yourself on bringing a spirit of peace to people in conflict? Bring peace. Whatever it is that you most cherish about how you wish to live your life, it is the connection and expression of those qualities that help you to be centered and grounded. When you are centered and grounded, your presence with people... and the spirit that you bring to your work... will be palpably different from when you are not. When you are really present with people, you are already providing good, foundational, spiritual care.

The clinical arena: Connecting with what matters to your patients

For most of us, our clinical work with people in health and wellness care is the focus of our professional mission. We may bring a variety of personal motivations to our work… a curiosity for science, a passion for leadership, a desire for financial stability, a joy in a camaraderie of caregivers… but ultimately, the work we do is focused on healing suffering people and fostering wellness and wholeness in all of us.

We will consider approaches to spiritual care in the clinical arena in considerable detail. The common theme or direction of these approaches is supporting people on their own unique spiritual journeys by helping them to connect with what matters most to them. Where does the patient in front of you find meaning and purpose? What is her life "about?" What does he hope the legacy of his life would be? What does she consider sacred? What is he really passionate about? What sustains her in hard times? Answers to such questions, as we shall see, provide a vital backdrop for patients' choices about health practices, a template for patients' charting the places where they will invest their time and heart, and a wellspring of wisdom and direction in adversity.

The organizational arena: Connecting with the shared energy of people working together

Organizations have souls as much as people do. Organizational soul comes by a variety of names; "spirit," "atmosphere," "culture," "tone," "environment," and so forth. Some organizations "have it," some do not, and the difference is usually palpable.

I suspect that you have experienced (or perhaps heard from other people) about great places to work, and experienced (or heard from others) about places where work was pretty demoralizing. Practicing in and living near the state capital of Maine, I have known a large number of state employees over the years and heard their stories about work. Occasionally I hear about state departments where people really believe in what they are doing… protecting a watershed, preserving a historic past, providing educational services for teenage mothers… and work together with a spirit of respect, support and joy. I hear of other state departments or units where people are predominantly putting in their time until they are fully vested in the retirement system, and where the workplace spirit seems to nurture suspicion, micromanaging, backbiting, and protecting one's own turf. Clearly, the former group of departments will support the health and well-being of employees better than the latter group, and I would bet a pair of Red Sox tickets that the former group of departments would show much better indices of productivity and organizational functioning, as well.

There is, in fact, very substantial literature in the business community about the relationship between organizational spirit and parameters of organizational functioning and success. One of the very early books in this area was "The Soul of a Business" by Tom Chappell, a narrative of the history and evolution of Tom's of Maine, the organic personal care products company that Chappell founded with his wife, Kate.[2] Starting from their home in Kennebunk, Maine, the Chappells built a business that was profitable but, by the late 1970s, had reached a plateau. Tom believed that something was missing, and he negotiated with his board to drop back to half time and to devote the remainder of his time to studying theology at Harvard Divinity School.

He had a blast, studying Martin Buber, Jonathan Edwards and other spiritual writers, and bringing back to Maine a new energy for integration of spiritual wisdom and consciousness in business practice. With his board, he then revisited the kind of organization they wished to lead, in terms of empowerment of employees, stewardship of the environment, and substantial engagement with the local community. The results of this undertaking, from a purely business standpoint, were striking.

So, too, in health care. There are good data in this arena, as well, as we will review. The short summary is that health care organizations that pay attention to organizational soul… a shared sense of mission, respect and empowerment of employees, a spirit of community and caring among workers… do better than organizations that do not with respect to employee retention and satisfaction, patient satisfaction, performance improvement and process measures, and health care outcomes.

Three interlocking pieces

I believe that all three arenas are vital parts of the larger picture of spirituality in health and wellness care. Spiritual care is incomplete without attention to personal spirituality, as well as clinical approaches, as well as organizational soul. Take one in isolation… a common example being good clinical skills in dis-spirited practitioners or disempowering organizations… and the challenges of providing good spiritual care over time become formidable and prohibitive.

Stated positively, the possibilities of providing good spiritual care can be exciting in the setting of centered and grounded practitioners, with solid and practical clinical approaches, in organizations that empower staff and patients alike to bring out the best that is within them.

I tell participants in my workshops that 92 percent of the literature on spirituality and health care addresses the clinical arena, 7.5 percent of the literature addresses the personal arena, with a scattering of publications addressing the organizational arena. I confess that I am making these numbers up, but I suspect that they would come close to the actual emphasis in each of these three arenas.

In the main body of this book, we will consider each of these arenas in detail, exploring what they are, why they matter, how they interrelate, and how they may be nurtured.

POSITIVE SPIRITUALITY

What is "positive spirituality?" Is some spirituality "negative?" What does "Positive Spirituality in Health Care" mean?

Good questions. Thanks for asking.

Consider; a parent anguishes over why a loving God would visit a three year old child with cancer. A man dying of AIDS struggles to reconcile his homosexuality with his lifelong devotion to the Catholic Church. A middle-aged woman is drawn into a sexual relationship with her pastor... which she ends... and faces challenges of forgiveness and trust.

These are serious spiritual issues; challenges that call into question people's core spiritual values about themselves, the world and, indeed, the nature of the Divine. I think that clinicians in health and wellness care can work with people around issues like these to a lesser or greater extent depending on a number of factors, such as our skills and experience, our comfort level, and the kinds of ongoing relationships we have had. Often, however, people struggling with issues such as these can be best served by spiritual care professionals such as chaplains, spiritual directors and clergy.

"Positive spirituality" complements the journey of identifying and healing spiritual issues. Positive spirituality comes at spirituality from the other direction. The question is not "What is wrong?" The question is "What is right?" The question is not primarily how spiritual suffering and spiritual wounds can be healed; the question is more one of identifying and encouraging people's spiritual values and resources, and bringing those values and resources to bear in people's journeys toward health, coping, dignity and wellness.

The positive spirituality conversation takes shape along lines I have described above, and will explore in considerable detail.

- *What is your life about?*
- *What matters to you?*
- *What do you care about?*
- *What is sacred for you; what do you cherish?*

- *What sustains you and keeps you going in adversity?*
- *What are the qualities of character that you most take pride in and try to express in your life?*

As I write this, I saw a patient this week for the first time, who described a lifelong history of abuse and mental health issues. She began the conversation with a recitation of the various psychiatric diagnoses she had accumulated... PTSD, depression, bipolar disorder, and borderline personality disorder... and then proceeded to describe the terrible physical and sexual abuse that had been visited upon her by her father over a number of years. She had had multiple suicide attempts, the most recent three years ago upon the death of a cherished grandfather. One could feel and see the weight of this suffering in her telling the story.

It occurred to me to confirm with her that she had indeed not attempted suicide in the last three years... this was the case... and to ask why. For much of this time, she said, she had been engaged in caring for her widowed grandmother, spending time with her and helping her with her own health problems, until the grand-mother passed away, as well. Did my patient think that her caring for the grandmother had anything to do with her refraining from suicide attempts during this time? Yes, she believed that it did. How would she put into words what it was about caring for the grandmother that helped her to remain on this side of suicide? She paused,

I think it gave me a purpose in my life, a purpose for being on this planet.

We spoke more about the idea of "purpose" and how that had made a difference in her life; one could see and feel the weight of the suffering diminishing. This is "positive spirituality."

Of course, she has some significant spiritual issues to address. How do you deal with years of sexual abuse at the hands of someone who should be a champion and protector? What does "forgiveness" mean and how might this at some point be a part of the journey?

Important questions; genuine spiritual issues. But it is clear that she is more than the person who has been terribly victimized. She is also a person who has a heart of tenderness for aging grandparents, and who has made the profoundly important connection that "purpose for being on this planet" can be a vital part of her own healing journey.

Positive spirituality, in other words, affirms that people may have substantial spiritual issues and suffering, but directs energy particularly toward the spiritual values and resources that sustain and empower people as they live their lives.

As a practical matter, what I am calling spiritual "issues" and spiritual "resources" often intersect. You see both in the brief story I have told about my abused patient. We will touch on the subject of spiritual issues and suffering and consider some approaches for providers of health and wellness care, while the over-arching theme of the following chapters will be the understanding and nourishment of spiritual values and resources, in personal, clinical and organizational venues.

A LOOK FORWARD

The first three chapters of this book provide background material for a clinically-oriented perspective on spirituality and spiritual care. Chapter 1 presents some definitions and perspectives about spirituality, including an introduction to my CAMPS framework for exploring five dimensions of spiritual experience. Chapter 2 describes four reasons why spirituality is important in health and wellness care. Chapter 3 considers the nature of spiritual care, and how health and wellness care clinicians can provide great spiritual care, in partnership with spiritual care specialists. Chapter 4 examines the three arenas of spiritual care... personal, clinical and organizational... in greater detail.

The main body of the book presents nine chapters that explore the "Nine Practical Approaches to Pursuing Wholeness for Clinicians, Patients and Health Care Organizations." Chapters 5 through 7 consider the *personal* arena of spiritual care, exploring personal purpose, positive qualities of character, and healing intention and presence. Chapters 8 through 10 consider the *clinical* arena of spiritual care, exploring spiritual inquiry, partnering with patients in pursuing what they care about, and recurring themes of transcendence and valued directions. Chapters 11 through 13 consider the *organizational* dimension of spiritual care, exploring organizational mission and values, organizations as "community," and empowering leadership.

Sprinkled throughout are twenty-four practical strategies for building on the ideas and case examples we will be considering. You may also think of these strategies as "exercises," or suggestions for "active learning."

Finally, two appendices present a dozen or so helpful websites about spirituality and health, and A Fiddler's Dozen of Fred's Favorite Books on Spirituality and Health Care.

May this book affirm the heart and the skill that you already bring to your work, and may we explore together some additional approaches to supporting people on their journeys toward healing and wholeness.

REFERENCES

1. Myss C. Invisible acts of power. In: Church D, ed. *Healing the Heart of the World*. Santa Rosa, CA: Elite; 2005:17-21.
2. Chappell T. *The Soul of a Business*. New York: Bantam; 1993.

The Context

Chapter One

Perspectives on Spirituality

*The spiritual is inclusive. It is the deepest
sense of belonging and participation.
We all participate in the spiritual at all times, whether we know it or not.
There's no place to go and be separated from the spiritual... The most
important thing in defining spirit is the recognition that the spirit
is an essential need of human nature. There is something in all of us
that seeks the spiritual. This yearning varies in strength from person to
person but it is always there in everyone.
And so, healing becomes possible.[1]*

Rachel Naomi Remen, MD

Some time during the second half of the first century of the
Common Era, a fisherman and missionary in Asia Minor contrasted
spiritual and material pursuits. According to John the Apostle, as
he is known in the Christian tradition, "It is the spirit who gives
life; the flesh profits nothing. The words I have spoken to you are
spirit and are life" (NIV).

The modern literature on spirituality and human experience
offers countless perspectives on spirituality. At its core, however,
I am drawn to the idea that spirit gives life. Spirit... however

you think of this and from whatever tradition you come… gives meaning, dignity, direction and passion to life.

As I speak with people about spirituality, I often hear a connection between being spiritually engaged and being fully and meaningfully alive:

T.S. was a 34 year old female who complained of a complete loss of libido. At the time of presentation the insufferable complaint had been going on for greater than 3 years without any improvement. Over the course of two years her complaint was not found to be secondary to a hormonal imbalance, an anatomical condition, any metabolic or organic problem, or a primary depression. Psychotherapy, couples counseling, and sensate focus were also tried unsuccessfully. Some time later, I had the opportunity to follow-up with her and she had finally experienced a resolution of her symptoms after 5-6 years of suffering. She explained that she had come to realize that several life events had occurred simultaneously that had left her feeling "spiritually dead" and completely detached from her spiritual self and the "experience of God" that she had always known. Apparently, she was not able to realize this previously and no amount of talking or suggestions had led to her reconnecting with her spiritual self. She began her journey of healing after listening to an audio-tape on intuition and love. A suggestion was made to experience getting in touch with all of her senses through self-guided imagery. She began to re-awaken and also began nurturing herself through nature and rest while creating experiences to connect with her senses. Eventually this exploration allowed her to redefine a sense of spiritual connection and "being present" in her life. This allowed her to feel whole again and spiritually alive. Her libido followed.

In the framework of this patient, there is a clear distinction drawn between being spiritually "dead" and spiritually "alive," and this distinction has profound implications for her health and for the ways that she lives her life.

The last eighteen or twenty years have witnessed a substantial increase in the interest in spirituality and health care. When I presented a seminar about spirituality at a Society of Teachers of Family Medicine national conference in 1986,[2] and when I published (with the late David Larson) what I believe was the first article about spirituality in the Family Medicine literature in 1988,[3] there was clearly a feeling that people interested in this subject were part of a small, ragtag band outside of the mainstream of organized medicine.

How much has changed in the intervening years. One can go to STFM conferences these days and find that seminars and interest group conversations about spirituality consistently spill out into the halls. Thanks to the efforts of Dr. Larson, Dr. Christina Puchalski (Founder and Director of the George Washington Institute for Spirituality and Health), the Templeton Foundation, and many others, there are now educational curricula about spirituality at a majority of American medical schools, a number of postgraduate programs, and at least one program (several fellowships in Integrative Medicine at the Arizona Center for Integrative Medicine) addressed to mid-career physicians. Dr. Herbert Benson's Harvard conference on Spirituality and Healing in Medicine has been packing them in for many years. The number and quality of research projects about the incorporation of spirituality in health care has increased substantially, as we shall see later, and there have been significant research initiatives (sponsored by the Fetzer Institute, among others) in a number of ancillary subject areas such as forgiveness, gratitude, hope, and love. And at a personal level, I talk about this subject with medical students who are applying to our residency program and find lively and engaged interest, in contrast to the quizzical and worried expressions of years past.

Still, there is much more work to be done, and many questions remaining to be explored. What is the larger picture... what does it mean to incorporate spirituality in health care? Where are the points in patients' lives and in the process of health care where conversation about spirituality may be helpful? How do we best enter this arena with patients? How can we best approach spirituality in an inclusive and respectful way with our patients? As we encounter or elicit spiritual issues in our relationships with patients, what do we as providers of health and wellness care *do?* What is our unique role… as physicians, nurses, acupuncturists, naturopaths, psychologists, physical therapists, medical assistants and others in the health care world… in strengthening patients' spiritual resources and ameliorating spiritual suffering? How can we best collaborate with pastoral care professionals, drawing on their skills and expertise and also being legitimate players in this arena ourselves? How is our own spirituality related to what we do as health care professionals?

PERSPECTIVES ON SPIRITUALITY

What do we mean by "spirituality?" Why do we speak of "spirituality," rather than "religion?" What is the relationship of spirituality and religion? Does reference to "spirituality" imply a particular world view?

Good questions, all. It would certainly be sensible to lay out a clear definition of spirituality, as we embark on an exploration of spirituality and health care.

This is, however, not so easy. My observation is that the word "spirituality" rolls frequently and smoothly off the tongue, but takes on a broad variety of meanings to different people. If you tell me that spirituality is an important part of your life, I may make some assumptions about your having some cherished values or beliefs, or perhaps assume that you engage in some centering or grounding practices. But I would be guessing… and I would certainly need to have a conversation with you about this before I began to have some real appreciation of what this meant to you.

For me, the most succinct statement of the overarching picture of spirituality comes from former Surgeon General Dr. C. Everett Koop. Speaking in 1994 at the annual Maine symposium on spirituality and health that I coordinate, he defined spirituality as

The vital center of a person; that which is held sacred.[4]

Along with the observation from John the Apostle, I think that this points to themes that can be profoundly helpful as we care for patients. What is "the vital center" for a middle aged man who has had a serious heart attack? What sustains a grade school teacher who feels overwhelmed and depressed? What is sacred enough for a young mother to energize her efforts to stop smoking? When are the times when a retired person feels really alive? What keeps a high school student who has had suicidal ideas from carrying them out? When, indeed, do we experience something sacred in our professional lives? What sustains and re-orients us when we become overextended and demoralized?

As we understand… for our patients and for ourselves… what "gives life" and what is "vital and sacred," we glimpse the foundation that underlies the personal meaning of health and wholeness. We understand better the personal nature of suffering. We understand better the personal motivation for change. And we are given the opportunity and the honor of engaging the personally-understood life force that sustains all of us as people on our life journeys.

DEFINING SPIRITUALITY

Before we consider further the "content" of spirituality… the aspects of human experience that this broad word embraces… I would like to suggest several ideas about the process of approaching a definition.

Spirituality is personal

Spirituality is uniquely experienced and understood by individual people.

There may be common beliefs and practices among groups of people, but ultimately the understanding of what is vital and sacred is uniquely our own. Mennonites may share beliefs about adult baptism. Southern Baptists may share beliefs about the literal interpretation of biblical texts. Hasidic Jews may express their faith in common ways in terms of ritual and celebration. Participants in Alcoholics Anonymous may embrace together the convention of referring to a "Higher Power." Activists with the Nature Conservancy may orient much of their personal and professional lives around sustaining the natural environment. But in each of these cases, an articulation of what is vital and sacred… what gives life… will be in the unique language, drawing on the unique personal experiences, of individual people.

Indeed, any definition of spirituality is itself a personal matter. I am suggesting some core ideas about spirituality that make sense to me, and I will shortly be suggesting several common aspects of spiritual experience. I do this not so much because I think there is a right way to think about spirituality, but because a) I think I owe it to readers to let you know where I am coming from, and b) because much of what I will be describing about how I work with spirituality with patients and health professionals follows from my understanding of spirituality.

In practice, I find that most people who would care to define spirituality have their own definition, and have some emotional attachment to this definition. I would rather honor the framework and language of people's personal definitions, rather than impose my own. Honoring the unique definition of "spirituality" held by individual people is respectful of them, and empowering as they cultivate and pursue what is vital and sacred for them.

Spirituality as experience

Spirituality is, first, experienced. It is secondarily put into words.

I love models and frameworks and paradigms. It warms my heart to draw boxes and arrows that depict directions of influence among aspects of human experience. But the clearest pathway to understanding the spiritual dimension of someone's life is not found in seeking the words, but in seeking the experiences. As we will consider when we examine spiritual inquiry, a question such as, "When has there been a time when you have experienced something really sacred and powerful in your life?" typically yields a much more rich and substantial response than asking people about their theology or belief systems.

I have had two good friends and colleagues, ages 46 and 55, die of cancer in the last couple of years. Both of them, until the very end, were among the most "vital" and "alive" people I have known... caring about other people, learning and growing, cherishing their days. One spoke comfortably in spiritual language; one did not. Neither one needed to speak formally about their spirituality. You could see it. You could feel it.

Spirituality as narrative

More specifically, the richness of spirituality often resides in stories.

A few years ago, I did a qualitative research project that involved interviewing family physicians about what "spirituality" meant to them and how they incorporated it into their professional and personal lives.[5] The subjects were 12 physicians from three regions of the country. Six were male and six female. They were all either in full-time clinical practice, or had had substantial clinical practice experience. All were referred to me because intervening contacts thought that they would have an interest in talking about spirituality and medicine. They were involved, to a greater or lesser extent, with a broad variety of spiritual communities, reflecting both Western and Eastern traditions.

I spoke with all of them about their experiences and perspectives about spirituality and medicine, then processed the interview transcripts according to a typical content analysis methodology. The results were striking both for what these physicians did not talk about and what they did talk about.

These physicians did not much speak about religion, spiritual history-taking, chaplains, or spiritually-related techniques such as prayer and meditation. Rather, they told rich and touching stories of patients' struggles, courage, determination and really coming to grips with issues of what it means to live, and to die. They told stories, as well, about their own lives and, often, what it meant to them to be doctors and healers.

I had a fellow who started seeing me for some sinus problems and back problems. As I began to get to know him, he kind of opened up a little and said that his son had been killed in an auto accident about a year or two before. We talked a little bit about it and he kind of closed off the discussion and I wrapped up the medical things and gave him a prescription and he went on.

He came back again about a month later. He was having more back problems and some stress situation reactions. We talked again and I asked him how he was feeling. Was he depressed at all? And how he was dealing with the fact of losing his son? So that gave us the opportunity again to talk a little bit more about that. And he broke down. He said he thought he had begun to turn a corner, but it was still really hard.

He just cried and said, "It was the worst thing I ever had to deal with. I was depressed and I really wanted to kill myself." I said, "Well, what has started to make a difference?"

And he said, "The last time you talked to me, you know, you were so concerned about how I was doing… I felt like you really understood what it was like to go through what I'd been going through. I remember you asked what I was doing for myself… was I exercising, was I seeing friends, had I been going to church, and things like that. After that, my wife and I sat down and talked. I turned on the TV to one of the religious programs and we listened and we started doing those things again. It's really made a difference in my life."

Over the next few months, he got a job at Ignatius house, which is the AIDS program here in town. He put his heart into that and really started talking with those fellows about how they were doing, too. He said it's made a difference. We got him into counseling. He's gone back to church. Stopped alcohol, stopped the meds he'd been taking. I really have seen a big change in his life. It's not like I deserve the credit for all of this, but I think I may have had a role in caring about him and encouraging him about the things that might help him to bring his life back together.

Most healing traditions are deeply rooted in narrative and story-telling. Even in Western medicine, we typically begin our conversation about people with stories: "I have a 47 year old bank manager who was working in his garden Thursday when he experienced a sharp pain...". As we hear (and participate in) patients' stories, spirituality "comes alive" and engages the listener. Something happens to us personally and spiritually as we hear people's stories of pain, suffering, courage, determination and commitment.

Spirituality as "embodiment," rather than "specialty"

Spirituality in health care subsumes, but is not defined by, specific techniques and approaches.

We will consider in the next chapter a substantial research literature on the relationships between spiritual and religious beliefs and practices and health. Much of this research looks at the beneficial effects of a variety of observable behaviors and spiritual techniques... religious institution attendance, prayer and meditation, spiritual assessment, chaplain consultation, and so forth. As we work with patients, we try to understand and support the spiritual practices that have been helpful to patients, and to find concrete spiritual resources that have been helpful to us.

While we embrace such techniques and approaches in working with patients, however, I believe that the definition of spirituality in health care is broader than techniques and approaches. An integrative approach to thinking about spirituality has its roots in the ways in which spirituality informs who we are as people and practitioners, and how spirituality informs the mission and culture and spirit of the organizations of which we are a part. It has its roots in the larger picture of how "the spiritual" is embodied, and given life, in the experience of patients and in ourselves. For a patient with metastatic cancer, coming to an understanding of what life will be about and what is "vital and sacred" during their remaining time is the larger picture. The techniques we use, such as prayer, meditation or religious participation can be viewed as methodologies in service to this larger picture.

The "landscape" of spirituality, in other words, is large. Specific techniques and approaches dot the landscape, but do not define the whole picture.

The specialty model. I have proposed two contrasting perspectives on the larger picture of spirituality in health care; the "specialty" model and the "embodiment" model.[6] What I call the "specialty model" views spirituality as a specific content area, or area of technical expertise, in parallel with countless other content areas (such as cardiology and ENT) that health care practitioners need to make a part of their repertoire. Primary care physicians, for instance, operate from a variety of specialty areas as the clinical situation warrants. Sometimes they may "do" cardiology in working with a patient with heart disease. Sometimes they may "do" neurology, or gastroenterology, or orthopedics. At other times, they do not engage these specialty areas. There is not much need for a textbook of Internal Medicine when doing a well-child exam, for instance.

In the "specialty model," spirituality is incorporated in the process of health care in the same way as any other specialty content area; sometimes you "do it" and sometimes you don't. In this model, certain clinical situations (such as death and dying or profound disability) lead health care practitioners to shift into a "spirituality mode" and engage this particular content area with specific techniques and approaches. Practitioners may conduct an organized spiritual assessment, recommend prayer, teach meditation, and so forth. Apart from clinical situations that trigger the spirituality mode, spirituality content is put away, just as one keeps the Medicine textbook on the shelf during the pediatric exam.

The embodiment model. We may contrast the "specialty" way of thinking about spirituality with what I call the "embodiment model." In the embodiment model, spirituality lies at the core of what it means to be a provider of health care, acting as an agent of healing in people's lives.

Spirituality is embodied in everything we do. The work that we do as health care practitioners is informed and guided by how we see ourselves and how we come to understand and give life to our sense of vocation, calling and mission.

No matter what the content area, there is a spirit in the room as we work with patients… which we can feel and experience, even if it can't be adequately put into words. We may try, perhaps with some success, to capture this spirit with a variety of words… *calm, compassionate, time-urgent, businesslike, welcoming, honoring, analytical, detached,* and so forth.

We will consider later some of the literature on "presence" and "intention" in health care. The thrust of this literature is that our spirits, or the ways in which spirit is visible or experienced in us as health care givers… matters. How spirit is embodied in the work we do, in other words, has a bearing on the healing process.

I have an elderly patient who has struggled for many months with the impending death of her sister from end stage CA. She always included a description (usually tearful) of how her sister was doing at her visits with me, as well as what it was like for her to experience her sister's decline. She was especially feeling helpless and guilty as the oldest sibling who'd been the one others would always look to for help in the past. At first I was uncomfortable as I felt something more was expected of me besides listening. However at subsequent visits I realized she just needed to tell her story. Even though the telling was not easy she always seemed lifted after and I could sense a deepening spiritual connection between us.

The term, "spiritual connection" signifies to me that a spirit of healing has been embodied in the person and presence of this practitioner. I would not be surprised if the patient were to describe this relationship with words like "respect" or "safety" or "compassion" or "caring" or even "love." It can perhaps be argued that what the practitioner is doing in this relationship is reducible to definable techniques such as active listening, or perhaps qualities of non-verbal behavior like optimal eye contact and physical distance. I don't doubt that behaviors and techniques at this level could be reliably identified on a videotape of office encounters with this patient, but my belief is that what is happening is not fully reducible to such component parts.

I often find, incidentally, that phrases like "I was just listening" in healing narratives tip us off that the embodiment of spirit in the practitioner has been a profoundly important part of the process.

Comparing/contrasting the models. The idea of "embodiment" is vitally important in how we think about what it means to provide spiritual care. We will consider further in later sections.

The distinction between specialty and embodiment is also significant in terms of health care education and program development.

My experience with primary care physicians is that when they reflect on the specialty model of spirituality, there is often a great sighing weariness about seeing *yet another* area of content and expertise to master. The operational word for the embodiment model, in contrast, is "already." Health care practitioners *already* understand, experience, appreciate, and embody these things... at least to some degree.

At some point, all of us have the experience of remembering why we went into health care, what it means to be a healer in somebody's life, and how we are enriched by the struggles, triumphs, and life experience of patients and colleagues with whom we work. The language and paradigm of what we as educators do in this area should not so much be "introducing" or "teaching" as it should be "developing" or "cultivating." We develop, cultivate and create conditions for the expression of that which is already there.

Spirituality is dynamic

Few of us, and few of our patients, remain at the same place spiritually across the life span.

I grew up a Catholic, but pretty much lost interest in religious life during college and medical school. Now that I have children, I'm interested in some religious grounding for them, although I think I have been too put off by the scandals in the Catholic Church to go back there. I guess I have also become broader as I have seen more of the world and learned more about different religious traditions. We go to a Protestant church now, but I think my own spirituality is partly that and partly Buddhist and maybe some other things too.

Defining spirituality is more a matter of recognizing a dynamic and emerging process, than looking at a static set of beliefs or practices.

Spirituality and religion

Finally, spirituality is not equivalent to religion.

For many people, answers to the questions of what is "vital" and "sacred" and "gives life" are answered within the context of particular religious traditions and values. For many people, they are not. For many other people, the approaches to these fundamental life questions are informed in some ways by religious values and traditions, but are also uniquely personal, as I have suggested above.

This distinction has been gradually emerging over the last generation. A remarkable series of studies by sociologist Wade Roof[7] shows that the Baby Boom generation in America is deeply spiritual, although in a very different way from their parents. The generation of people born between 1946 and 1964 partake of a "spiritual marketplace" which provides a broad range of resources to address what Roof describes as hunger for meaning, authenticity and intimate relationships. This generation shows much less connection to particular religious traditions and institutions than the generation preceding them.

Population studies suggest that Americans draw a distinction between spirituality and religion,[8] and tend to see spirituality as the broader concept.[9] There are also some data that suggest that medical patients make a distinction between spirituality and religiousness. A recent study of patients with serious medical illnesses, for instance,[10] found that 43% identified themselves as spiritual, 37% identified themselves as religious, and 20% as both. While similarities in beliefs and behavior were observed between the spiritual and religious groups, there were some significant differences. The spiritual group, for instance, tended to view God as more loving, forgiving and nonjudgmental, while the religious group perceived God as more of a judgmental creator.

So it is with epidemiological research about spirituality, as well. Much of the early research twenty or more years ago examined the associations of health status with denomination affiliation. Cancer incidence in Mormons. Heart disease incidence in Seventh Day Adventists. Religious observance and plasma lipids among Jewish residents of Jerusalem. This research has grown up over the years, looking at more sophisticated and multidimensional expressions of religiousness such as religious institution attendance, religious coping, self-rated religiousness and ratings of strength and comfort from religion.[11]

There is also a growing conversation in this epidemiological re-search about the distinction between spirituality and religion[12-14] and a growing number of measurement instruments that differ-entiate spirituality and religion,[15] focus exclusively on spirituality[16] and, indeed, do not make the presumption of theism.[17] We will examine these and other measurement approaches as we consider spiritual inquiry.

As I frequently tell groups, I don't want to diminish the often-profound importance of religious traditions, connections and values in human experience... but neither do I want to define spirituality in terms of religiousness.

SO WHAT, THEN, *IS* SPIRITUALITY?

You are concluding, by now, that I believe it is not useful to seek to craft a single, succinct, crisp, universal definition of spirituality. I think that the exercise of defining what this word means to any of us is probably more important than obligingly signing on to someone else's definition. The Koop definition ("the center of a person; that which is held sacred") is appealing to me as I work with people, and I will shortly propose several dimensions of spirituality that round out a picture of the types of human experience that I think this concept embraces. These perspectives may or may not appeal to you. I would invite you to take a few minutes to put into words your own understanding of spirituality, and to consider how your ideas may be informed by the issues we are considering.

For further reflection, let me give you some examples of how some mid-career physicians have defined spirituality for themselves. Following are some definitions from participants in the Fellowship Program at the Arizona Center for Integrative Medicine. As you will see, there are both common themes and a breadth of understanding.

Spirituality is tending to that which gives each of us our heart and soul.

It is about expanding beyond myself and connecting with what is larger... the mystery of life. Translating that connection into who I am and what I do, thereby living with meaning and purpose.

A recognition of love, which is the lifeline which flows through us all.

A feeling of being totally alive and vibrant. A feeling of connection to yourself and to the community and the universe.

I think that spirituality is an awareness of the life force that binds us together and which constantly reminds me that I was placed on this earth to do something unique and of consequence for others around me.

Spirituality is experiencing our vital positive essence and its relationship to others, our world and a higher power.

As I look at these perspectives, I see themes about spirituality as a life force, or a flow of energy or spirit. About a relationship with things larger than ourselves. About meaning and purpose. About what makes us uniquely human, and uniquely the people that we are. About being able to be where we are and partake of the richness of the life experience before us.

You can't *not* have it

A final note about perspectives. With the kinds of broad and inclusive perspectives about spirituality that we are considering, *you really can't not have a spiritual dimension to life,* in the same way that a family therapist once pointed out that you can't *not* communicate. People may or may not be engaged with a religious community, and people may or may not use spiritual language, but everyone has some "vital center." Everyone has some things that they hold sacred. Everyone has some times… that may or may not be related to their physical health status… when they are really alive.

I sometimes see case formulations that touch on different aspects of patients' lives and see the comment "none" for the category "spirituality." I believe that this is rarely, if ever, true. I think I have never seen a patient who could not respond in some way to questions (with appropriate language) such as:

- *What is the most important thing in your life?*
- *What do you think is the reason why you're here?*
- *What sustains you and keeps you going in the hard times?*
- *When have been some times when you have felt really alive?*
- *What are you passionate about?*
- *What beliefs do you have about a power or force beyond yourself?*
- *What do you take pride in?*
- *What would you wish to be remembered for?*

DIMENSIONS OF SPIRITUALITY

In addition to loving models and frameworks and paradigms, I love acronyms. I will always remember the seven symptoms of major depression, for instance, because of the cherished *sig-e-caps* acronym.

The world of spirituality and health care has its share of acronyms, as well. FICA,[18] HOPE,[15] and the SPIRITual history[19] are among the frameworks that aim to define the dimensions of spirituality and to provide a succinct mnemonic for clinical assessment.

As part of a grant I received in 2002 from the George Washington Institute for Spirituality and Health (supported by the John

Templeton Foundation), I developed the CAMPS framework for teaching our residents and faculty some approaches to spiritual assessment. I suppose we all have our individual ways of doing things, and it seemed to me that none of the other spiritual assessment frameworks captured quite what I want to be looking at as I think about patients' spirituality.

The name CAMPS is a little tongue in cheek. In Maine, "camps" is the name for those places that many of our fellow citizens go to nurture their spirituality by hunting, fishing and drinking beer... or, for that matter, just getting out in the Great North Woods. Particularly in the late Fall, developing frostbite and hypothermia by day and being warmed by a wood stove in an uninsulated structure by night has a way of restoring one's soul.

We will return to this framework in later chapters as we consider why spirituality is important and as we consider personal and professional applications of spirituality. For now, let me describe each of the five dimensions.

Community

"Community" refers to that dimension of spirituality that has to do with participation in supportive groups of people.

Perhaps there are exalted and highly-developed souls out there who can live out their spirituality totally absent of other people. There are certainly some historical examples of people like this, such as the desert fathers (and mothers) of the ninth century and the Irish monks who lived out their days in rude stone huts on the Aran Islands. Most of us, though, need meaningful social relationships as a context for living out what is vital and sacred in our lives. We need connections with other people to define what our lives are about, and to give expression to what our lives are about.

The key word is "meaningful." Relationships are meaningful when there is genuine knowing and being-known, and when there is interaction around something that matters. I think the common phrase, "kindred spirits" captures well this element of spirituality-as-community. Kindred spirits are people that we connect with where there is a sense that "we are in it together," and that there is some overlap in our personal journeys.

Quality is more important than quantity. We may regularly see a gas station attendant, or a co-worker, or the person who stakes out the seat next to us at church… but not have any meaningful relationships with these people. On the other hand, people with whom we have fairly limited contact in terms of venue and clock time can be important sources of community. My wife (who has the kind of disarming and engaged presence that gives her the reputation in our family for being able to find out strangers' life stories in about five minutes) interacts several times a week with the clerks at the rural post office where we have a box. There is almost never any contact outside of this setting, but clearly there is an element of community for her and for them. They keep current about families and interests and activities, they exchange recipes for bean soup and chicken spread, and there is a genuine spirit of gladness and caring in their relating to each other.

Community can be formal or informal. Religious organizations, of course, provide a meaningful source of community for many people. Churches, synagogues and other faith-based groups are places where many of us find kindred spirits. In the Christian tradition, Paul of Tarsus frequently uses the phrase "one another" in his letters to early churches to describe the qualities of relationships that should characterize communities of believers. "Belonging to one another." "Teach and admonish one another." "Love one another."

It is important to recognize, however, that people do not necessarily seek or find community in religious organizations. In the mainline Protestant community with which I am familiar, it is entirely possible to show up for years and not really to know or be known by other participants.

Countless organizations that are not expressly religious provide meaningful sources of community, as well. Alcoholics Anonymous. The Audubon Society. Political parties. Habitat for Humanity. The American Legion. The local school board. Neighborhood associations. Bridge clubs. Garden clubs. The Lions, Eagles, Odd Fellows, Moose, Masons, Rotary, Order of the Eastern Star and other service organizations. Men's groups. Women's groups. The coaches and officials of your local Little League. In rural Maine, the Grange. In organizations such as these, people have a commitment to come together for a shared purpose, and there is the opportunity for community.

Community can be informal, as well. I have friends who for years have been hosting a weekly Sunday night potluck dinner for any among a group of friends who happen to be available. My own experience is that I have been playing pickup basketball for many years with a fairly constant group of other men. Clearly at this point, in our forties and fifties, most of us are not in it for the athletic glory, but more because we know and are known by each other.

Increasingly, the workplace serves as a vital source of community for many people. In his recent book about spirituality and work, Jay Conger[20] makes the point that most of us spend more hours at the workplace than any other single setting in our lives, and that our relationships there often take greater importance than they did a generation ago because of the disconnectedness of families and the decline of organized religious participation.

I recently conducted a study of exemplary primary care practices in Maine, identifying and examining two community health centers that a group of nominators judged as exceptional in terms of clinical care, work environment, and group spirit.[21] A qualitative analysis of interview and field observation data revealed a number of categories and themes that served to understand why these practices are such great places to be an employee or a patient. A recurring theme had to do with caring relationships among staff, which many people described in terms of "community" and "family." Some examples:

"Community" is an appropriate term... being part of a group working with patients and families, and working and living in a community where you feel comfortable. (Receptionist)

I think staff are here because they really want to be. We have a good sense of community, people that care about each other. We have a job to do, but we enjoy it. (Physician)

The way people relate to me here makes me feel that I'm not only here to provide a service, but that I'm here because I fit, because I'm wanted. (Psychologist)

We're all very close, and we're all friends, in spite of having our ups and downs. We're close enough so we can feel each other's pain, you can see it in their eyes. You just make a point of giving a hug... and everybody here is not afraid of doing that. (Practice Manager)

People enjoy coming here to work. Even when hard things are happening for us personally, we find respite in work. It's not because it numbs your mind, but because it's a home, a place of solace. (Physician)

We especially look for caring when we want to hire somebody, because in order to be caring for the people you're working for, like your patients, you have to care for the people you work with. (Receptionist)

The volume of our work doesn't get in the way of the spirit here; the spirit is what allows us to do what we do. If I'm feeling overwhelmed, someone will rubbing my shoulders and doing what they can to help me get the work done. (LPN)

We really are like a family. We know each other really well and work well together. You can read if someone's having a bad day without even asking... you can tell that they are, just by their body language, just looking. You touch them on the back and say "you doing ok?" That kind of stuff happens often, and that's what makes it a wonderful place to work. (Social Services)

Finally, many of us find meaningful community in the context of family. In spite of the geographic dispersion of families compared with earlier generations, the connections we have with our kinfolk frame what we find vital and sacred in our lives. Indeed, when I speak with patients about what is important to them ("What are your highest priorities?" "What really matters to you?" "What has kept you going throughout your illness?" "What has kept you from acting on your suicidal ideas?"), I most frequently hear answers that have to do with family. "My relationship with my wife." "My sister… we've always been there for each other." "My grandchildren… I really want to be a good influence for my grandchildren."

And, of course, many of us and many of the people we work with *do not* find meaningful community in the context of family. It is a continuing source of sadness for me in my practice to hear the recurring stories of people who have been cut off, marginalized, demeaned and abused by family.

Activities

"Activities" refers to that dimension of spirituality that has to do with spiritually related activities and practices that provide coherence and comfort.

Included among spiritually related activities are disciplines, devotions, ceremonies, sacraments and rituals. There is sometimes an instrumental quality of spiritual activities, when people will report pursuing these practices in order to bring about certain results, such as peacefulness, centeredness and spiritual grounding. Sometimes spiritual activities are not linked to results at all, such as when religious adherents will engage in prayer or praise not in order to bring about specific outcomes, but because they believe these activities are simply expressions of their faith commitment.

A very helpful resource for understanding and following spiritual activities is a short book by Quaker theologian Richard Foster called "Celebration of Discipline."[22] Originally published in the late seventies, Foster's book has been updated and reprinted many times in the intervening years. He is writing about spiritual activities, which he describes as "disciplines," and divides them into three broad classes. "Inward disciplines" include meditation, prayer, fasting, and study. "Outward" disciplines include simplicity (choosing, as a disciplinary practice, to live humbly and simply), solitude, submission, and service. "Corporate" disciplines include confession, guidance, worship, and celebration.

All of these practices, Foster argues, serve to put people "in the way of God." For people who are not theistically inclined as Foster is, the concept is readily transferable... in the sense of spiritual activities that help people to connect with whatever vital and life-sustaining spirit or force that frames their understanding of the world.

Spiritual activities may draw upon traditions that date back centuries or millennia, such as communion and anointing rituals in the Christian community and Sabbath observances in the Jewish community. Ceremonies and rituals may also be created fresh as a way of centering or drawing upon spiritual energy in the midst of our modern, current life circumstances. Physicians Carl Hammerschlag and Howard Silverman offer fascinating examples and principles about how people have created meaningful rituals and ceremonies as part of their journeys toward personal health, well-being, and wholeness.[23]

The "activity" dimension of spirituality is also particularly enriched by cross-cultural perspectives and traditions. We in the West can certainly learn from a host of Eastern traditions... yoga, Qigong, Sufi water ceremonies... as well as practices that come from our own Native American community. I recently participated, for instance, in a Native American sweat lodge ritual. The sweat lodge is a centuries-old tradition (which was, ironically, banned in this country by the Bureau of Indian Affairs until the late 1970's) of purification, prayer and healing. Glowing hot stones from an outside fire are rolled into the lodge and doused with water, while the leader orchestrates a series of stories, chants, songs and prayers. I found the spirit of community among participants to be palpable and, as a newcomer, was struck by the profound role of the physical environment... the burning of sweet grass and the all-enfolding heat and humidity. It occurred to me how little that we in our Western traditions draw upon tactile and physical dimensions of experience in our spiritual activities.

Meaning and Purpose

"Meaning and purpose" refers to that dimension of spirituality that has to do with a sense of coherence in life events, and with our engagement with life in ways that matter.

Issues of meaning and purpose are experienced at two levels. There is, first, the *meaning that we attribute* to life events. We humans have an intractable habit of searching for the significance and implications of the things that happen in our lives.

Why do we get sick? What does it mean about us... what does it mean about God, or about our view of the universe... that we get sick? Why does your 55 year old music teacher patient have ovarian cancer? How do we make sense of the death of a vibrant high school athlete in an automobile accident? What does it say about the universe that a boy grows up unwanted and abused? What is it that enables one person to recover miraculously from a stroke, while another does not? How will your colleague's third heart attack change who she is and how she lives her life? What does it say that an ostensibly less-deserving person is promoted, while an ostensibly more deserving person gets a humble buy-out and a personal escort out the door? What does it say about the universe that the longsuffering Cubs have not won a World Series since 1908 and came oh-so-close in 2003, only to lose in the league championship series in a horrifying way that could not have been scripted by Stephen King?

Often there is a fairly direct connection between meanings and attributions on one hand, and emotional and physical experiences on the other hand. The cognitive therapy movement,[24] for instance, long ago identified relationships between people's negative appraisals of themselves, their circumstances and their futures with experiences of depression and anxiety. Depressed patients tend to see themselves as defective and inadequate, tend to interpret ongoing experiences in negative ways, and tend to make negative predictions about the future. There is now a substantial research literature showing that working with patients on testing, changing and acting against such negative appraisals can have significant clinical benefit.

You may also recall the classic research from the Second World War in which civilians and soldiers with comparable traumatic injuries were compared with respect to pain and disability. It was observed that soldiers with specific non-lethal battle injuries had significantly less pain and disability than civilians who sustained comparable injuries in stateside events such as motor vehicle accidents. The explanation was that for the civilians, these injuries represented major traumas in otherwise "normal" lives, while for the soldiers, these injuries meant that they would survive the war, and they would be coming home.

As we will discuss when we consider clinical issues, it is often most helpful to explore the meanings that patients associate with life events… *why is this happening and what does this mean?*

Second, issues of meaning and purpose are experienced at the level of *life purpose.* Many readers will be familiar with the story of Viktor Frankl, the Austrian psychiatrist who was imprisoned in four concentration camps during the Holocaust, losing his parents and several other members of his family, along with manuscripts representing his life's work up to that point.[25] As an outgrowth of his own suffering, Frankl developed an approach to psychotherapy known as logotherapy. Logotherapy focuses the healing journey on the quest for personal meaning, which Frankl says is approached "by creating a work or doing a deed, by experiencing something or encountering someone, and by the attitude we take toward unavoidable suffering."

Frankl quotes the First Century BCE Palestinian sage Hillel the Elder:

It is a characteristic constituent of human existence that it transcends itself, that it reaches out for something other than itself… a man's heart is restless unless he has found, and fulfilled, meaning and purpose in his life.

Meaning sustains and heals. As I work with clients in my psychological practice, I often wonder if perhaps the most important contribution I make to their lives is to attempt to connect them with whatever helps them to find meaning, purpose and dignity in their lives. As I write this, I met earlier this week with a middle-aged man who suffered what he describes as a "nervous breakdown" several years ago, resulting in the eventual loss of his job and marriage, and the diagnosis of ongoing mental illness. He has shown great courage in re-creating his life… defining what is important and what is not important to him, developing new personal and career directions, and devoting himself to supporting other people who suffer in similar ways. As I reflected to him his obvious heartfelt quest to "make a difference in the world," he said… with much emotion and tears… that that was what kept him going day to day on his sometimes lonely and often challenging journey.

My opinion… and my observation… is that all people are endowed with unique gifts and capacities that they may use in service of meaning and purpose. These may be gifts of character, like kindness, generosity, equanimity, or perceptiveness. These may also be capacities or talents; being able to teach, inspire, challenge, play the piano, write, sculpt, crochet, cook great blueberry pies, or hit baseballs a long way. Identifying, nurturing and giving life to one's gifts and capacities, for many people, is a vital part of the spiritual journey.

Meaning and purpose may be found in any of a number of arenas in life. For many people, the quest for meaning focuses on family relationships. Many people in my practice say that they are sustained and motivated by the hope of being a caring and loving parent or grandparent. For some people, the quest for meaning focuses on community connections; the woman who runs a local food bank, the man who serves as an AA sponsor, the couple who together serve as stewards of a land trust.

Increasingly, there is great interest in the Management arena in the ways in which people find meaning and purpose in their work. Consultant Richard McKnight speaks of the powerful effect for organizations when they can be "gently helping individuals to discover their own uniqueness and to find ways of attaching it to some endeavor above and beyond themselves."[26]

Connecting with meaning and purpose in work is certainly important for us in the health care field. I have seen quite clearly, over the years, that health care professionals who maintain an awareness of "vocation" and "calling" in their work exude more vitality and joy… and probably are better agents of healing… than those who experience their work primarily as "a job."

And, of course, meaning and purpose may be found in one's relationships with The Divine. There is, for many of us… not just the solitary desert fathers/mothers and Aran Islands hermits we spoke of earlier… some inherent value in living in ways that are consistent with honored values and with the movement of the divine presence as we understand it.

Passions

"Passion" refers to that dimension of spirituality that has to do with experiencing joy, and with being excited, passionate and engaged with some aspects of life.

When we are passionate about something, we are enthusiastic. Our modern word "enthusiasm" is derived from the Greek *enthousiasmos/entheos*, signifying "inspired from God." It is as though there is a divine inspiration, or in-spiriting, to be engaged with some pursuit.

One can be inspired and passionate about causes, values, or organizations. People may be passionate about partisan politics, the peace movement, the preservation of the environment, the local Hospice, the local DARE program, or little league baseball.

One can also be inspired and passionate about all manner of personal and solitary pursuits. My father was a kindly and upbeat man who was engaged with life on many fronts, with particular passions for books, choral music, travel and railroads. His passion for railroads began as a young man in the 1920's, when he sent away for timetables and route maps for all of the major American railroads, and subsequently pored over the layout and pathways of the American railroad system. As he traveled, he was perennially exploring and taking pictures of passenger stations, freight yards, locomotives, rolling stock and trestles. After the demise of passenger rail, he sought out and rode on excursion trains. Well into his eighties, he could describe system routes quite clearly… "the main line of the Union Pacific… Chicago, Des Moines, North Platte, Cheyenne, Salt Lake… and branch lines connecting…"

In a clinical context, a family physician comments,

I think there's a lot of healing that happens just by connecting spiritually with people. It's not about what's in a pill or even the length of time that you spend with the person. It's finding the energy in them that wants to keep going—the musician that wants to keep playing or the athlete that wants to get back on the court, and the mother who loves to cook and wants to get her family back together for a big meal. Just connecting with the real life force in that person.

Clearly, passions that explicitly aim to make the world a better place tie in with spirituality by means of meaning and purpose, as we have discussed above. I would argue that "spirit" is present in more personal and private passions, as well. There is a palpable spirit about people who exude joy and enthusiasm and passion. It is as though these qualities put positive energy into the world. My observation is that this is beneficial both to the holders and to the beholders of the passion. As we will consider later, I therefore make it my practice clinically to learn about the passions of the people I work with… what they are excited about, what brings them joy, and what they are doing when they lose track of time.

Relationships with Spirit

This dimension of spirituality has to do with the awareness and communion with a divine or transcendent presence... our personal relationships with Spirit.

I saw a woman in my practice yesterday, a physician, who is finding it very distressing to be working in a health care practice that she describes as chaotic, unsupportive and dysfunctional. In additional to putting into practice the psychological coping approaches she has learned over the years, she says that she is sustained a lot by her private faith. She points out that she has a relationship with God. She prays that God would take charge of the situations that she finds challenging, and that somehow God's purposes may be advanced in the chaotic and sometimes demeaning interactions in which she finds herself. She entertains the possibility that there is some reason... some metaphysical reason... for her being there right now in her life. All of this is very meaningful for her, and is not necessarily related to any community context of her faith. Apart from her participation in religious organizations and activities, and apart from her relationships with fellow religious travelers, she is talking about her personal relationship with Spirit, to which she turns for strength and guidance.

I hear this often from people. The personal communion with a transcendent presence is extraordinarily common and, at least in my neck of the woods, does not seem necessarily related to religious participation. People do refer to this presence or spirit with a host of different names... God (or Goddess), Jesus, Higher Power, and the Man Upstairs, among them.

Several years ago, sociologist Melvin Pollner published some fascinating research about divine relations, social relations, and well-being.[27] Using data from a large general social survey, he explored the extent to which relationships with other people and reported relationships with "divine others" affected psychological well-being. Regression analyses revealed that divine relationships had significant effects on several measures of well-being (controlling for sociodemographic variables and church attendance)… in some cases, to a greater extent than the effects of people's relationships with real or concrete individuals.

There are some data, and certainly centuries of tradition, about the association of spirit-relationships and healing. In Western religious traditions, this work typically appears under the rubric of "prayer." As of the 2003 publication of an excellent review of spiritual healing by Jonas and Crawford, for instance, there had been 13 studies of the effects of distant intercessory prayer in clinical settings, with 46% showing statistically significant effects on at least one health outcome measure.[28] Included among these studies were two landmark projects that investigated the role of distant intercessory prayer with patients in coronary care units.[29, 30] With a total of over 1300 patients, these studies revealed a number of significant positive differences in CCU course and outcome for prayed-for patients, compared with patients receiving usual care.

In Eastern religious traditions and non-religious arenas, work on the association of spirit-relationships and healing is typically organized under the rubric of "energy" healing. Many world cultures presume the presence of "life energy," having various names, which can be felt but not seen. Illness is often understood to result from the inadequate cultivation, distribution or blockage of this life energy, with healing approaches aiming to gather, purify and effectively distribute this energy. The ancient Chinese tradition of Qigong (which has an enormous number of forms and styles), for instance, has a long regional legacy of effectiveness, and a growing base of empirical support with our own scientific models in such areas as cardiovascular, respiratory and immune function.[31]

While the traditions in the energy healing arena do not necessarily make the assumption of a divine or transcendent presence, they do share with Western traditions the belief that there is a force… that is not often well understood or captured by our scientific models... that can be cultivated or drawn upon for the benefit of healing. Our relationships with such a presence, or force, is a dimension of spirituality.

SUFFERING

Finally, as we consider perspectives on spirituality, a few words about suffering. People suffer when circumstances threaten or compromise things that matter to them in their lives. In the framework we have been considering, people suffer when circumstances... illness, relationship difficulties, misfortune... compromise "the vital center," and "what is held sacred." People suffer when circumstances compromise their **C**ommunity relationships, their spiritually related and renewing **A**ctivities, their experience of **M**eaning and purpose, their pursuit of **P**assions, and their relationships with **S**pirit.

A 55 year old man made his living as a traveling representative for a manufacturing company, driving long distances around Maine, visiting clients and servicing accounts. He found great pleasure in the ability to move freely around a beautiful landscape, and in his long-term collaborative relationships and friendships with the people whom he would visit on his rounds. Away from work, he had spent a number of years building a house on some land he owned, feeling pride in his ability to do much of the sophisticated and physically-demanding work himself. Then he sustained a back injury, eventually requiring surgery and leaving him with chronic pain and substantially compromised mobility. He found it physically intolerable to drive any distance in a car, and found that he was unable to continue much of the work he had been doing on his home. He suffered.

This man suffered not so much because of the physical pain and limitations per se, but because the circumstances of his injury and disability had cut him off from things that mattered to him in his life. His vocation and his avocation together had been sources of community, routine, meaning, and passion. The challenge for him, emotionally and spiritually, was how to restore the integrity and intactness of his spiritual well-being, within the context of his physical limitations.

Such is the nature of suffering. In the landmark journal article in this field… which is required reading for students who reflect together with me about spirituality in medicine… physician Eric Cassel proposes that suffering comes from challenges to the integrity of persons. For all of us, he argues, our personhood has a host of dimensions… a past, family ties, a cultural background, social roles, an ability to act and create, routines, a secret life, a perceived future and what he calls a "transcendent dimension."[32] When illness or misfortune challenge any of these personal dimensions that define and give life to who we are, we suffer.

This suffering is highly personal and linked to our own values. Living in the Kennebec watershed in central Maine and enjoying outdoor activities, I confess that I sometimes find it hard to take a graceful, Zen perspective on rainy summer days. During graduate school in Utah, however, I recall greeting a rainy October day with absolute exhilaration after a relentless summer of dry heat.

Macular degeneration will probably present greater suffering to someone whose passion is reading the *New York Times* than to someone whose passion is playing bluegrass fiddle (which is almost exclusively done by ear, rather than from sheet music). Arthritic changes affecting finger joints will probably present greater suffering to the fiddler than to the *Times* reader. We will explore the idea of suffering as a clinical issue further in Chapter 10.

SUMMARY

- Two points of departure for thinking about spirituality are
  o the observation from John the Apostle that spirit "gives life."
  o the definition from C. Everett Koop, MD of spirituality as "the vital center of a person; that which is held sacred."
- Considerations in defining spirituality include:
  o Spirituality is *personal:* it is uniquely experienced and un-

derstood by individual people.

o Spirituality is, first, *experienced.* It is secondarily put into words.

o Spirituality is often *narrative;* the richness of spirituality often resides in stories.

o Spirituality in health care subsumes, but is not defined by, specific techniques and approaches. At its core, spirituality in health care is more a matter of *"embodiment"* than "specialty."

o Spirituality is *dynamic;* few of us, and few of our patients, remain at the same place spiritually across the life span.

o Spirituality is *not the same as religion.* For some people, spirituality is expressed in religious beliefs and practices, while for other people, it is not.

o People can't *not* have a spiritual dimension to life; everyone has a "vital center" and things that they "hold sacred," whether or not they use spiritual language.

• The CAMPS framework of dimensions of spirituality includes:

o **C**ommunity: participation with kindred spirits in supportive groups of people.

o **A**ctivities: spiritually related activities and practices that provide coherence and comfort.

o **M**eaning and purpose: our engagement with life in ways that matter.

o **P**assions: experiencing joy, and being excited, passionate and engaged with some aspects of life.

o Relationships with **S**pirit: the awareness and communion with a divine or transcendent presence.

• People *suffer* when circumstances threaten or compromise things that matter to them in their lives… "the vital center," and "what is held sacred."

REFERENCES

1. Remen R. On defining spirit. *Noetic Sciences Review.* 1998(47):64.
2. Craigie FC, Jr., Mitchell H. The role of spiritual values in family teaching. Paper presented at: Society of Teachers of Family Medicine Conference on Working with Families; March 8, 1986; Amelia Island, FL.
3. Craigie FC, Jr., Liu IY, Larson DB, Lyons JS. A systematic analysis of religious variables in The Journal of Family Practice, 1976-1986. *J Fam Pract.* Nov 1988;27(5):509-513.
4. Koop CE. Spirituality and health. Paper presented at: Thomas Nevola, MD Symposium on Spirituality and Health; June 8, 1994; Augusta, ME.
5. Craigie FC, Jr., Hobbs RF, 3rd. Spiritual perspectives and practices of family physicians with an expressed interest in spirituality. *Fam Med.* Sep 1999;31(8):578-585.
6. Craigie FC, Jr. Spiritual caregiving by health care professionals. *Health Progress.* 2007;88(2):61-65.
7. Roof WC. *Spiritual Marketplace: Baby Boomers and the Remaking of American Religion.* Princeton: Princeton University Press; 2001.
8. Shahabi L, Powell LH, Musick MA, Pargament KI, Thoresen C, Williams D. Correlates of self-perceptions of spirituality in American adults. *Annals of Beh Med.* 2002;24:59-68.
9. Zinnbauer BJ, Pargament KI, Cole B, Rye MS, Butter EM, Belavich TG. Religion and spirituality: Unfuzzying the fuzzy. *J for the Sci Stud of Religion.* 1997;36:549-564.
10. Woods TE, Ironson GH. Religion and spirituality in the face of illness: How cancer, cardiac and HIV patients describe their spirituality/religiosity. *J Health Psychology.* 1999;4:393-412.
11. McCullough ME, Hoyt WT, Larson DB, Koenig HG, Thoresen C. Religious involvement and mortality: A meta-analytic review. *Health Psychol.* May 2000;19(3):211-222.
12. Miller RM, Thoresen C. Spirituality, religion and health: An emerging research field. *Am Psychologist.* 2003;58(1):24-35.
13. Boudreaux ED, O'Hea E, Chasuk R. Spiritual role in healing: An alternative way of thinking. *Primary Care; Clinics in Office Practice.* 2002;29(2).

14. Hill PC, Pargament KI, Hood RW, et al. Conceptualizing religion and spirituality: Points of commonality, points of departure. *J for the Theory of Soc Behaviour.* 2000;30:51-77.

15. Anandarajah G, Hight E. Spirituality and medical practice: Using the HOPE questions as a practical tool for spiritual assessment. *Am Fam Physician.* Jan 1 2001;63(1):81-89.

16. Hatch RL, Burg MA, Naberhaus DS, Hellmich LK. The Spiritual Involvement and Beliefs Scale. Development and testing of a new instrument. *J Fam Pract.* June 1998;46(6):476-486.

17. Peterman AH, Futchett G, Brady MJ, Hernandez L, Cella D. Measuring spiritual well-being in people with cancer: The Functional Assessment of Chronic Illness Therapy- Spiritual Well-Being Scale (FACIT-Sp). *Annals of Beh Med.* 2002;24(1):49-58.

18. Post SG, Puchalski CM, Larson DB. Physicians and patient spirituality: Professional boundaries, competency and ethics. *Annals Int Med.* 2000;132(7):578-583.

19. Maugans TA. The SPIRITual history. *Arch Fam Med.* Jan 1996;5(1):11-16.

20. Conger JA, ed. *Spirit at Work: Discovering the Spirituality in Leadership.* San Francisco: Jossey-Bass; 1994.

21. Craigie FC, Jr., Hobbs RF. Exploring the organizational culture of exemplary community health center practices. *Fam Med.* 2004;36(10):733-738.

22. Foster R. *Celebration of Discipline: The Path to Spiritual Growth.* San Francisco, CA: HarperSanFrancisco; 1988.

23. Hammerschlag C, Silverman H. *Healing Ceremonies: Creating Personal Rituals for Spiritual, Emotional, Physical and Mental Health.* New York: Perigree; 1997.

24. Beck A, Rush A, Shaw B, Emery G. *Cognitive Therapy of Depression.* New York: Guilford; 1979.

25. Frankl V. *Man's Search for Meaning.* Boston, MA: Beacon Press; 2006.

26. McKnight R. Spirituality in the workplace. In: Adams J, ed. *Transforming Work: A Collection of Organizational Transformation Readings.* Alexandria, VA: Miles River Press; 1984:139-153.

27. Pollner M. Divine relations, social relations, and well-being. *J Health Soc Behav.* 1989;30(1):92-104.

28. Jonas WB, Crawford CC. Science and spiritual healing: A critical review of spiritual healing, "energy" medicine, and intentionality. *Alt Therapies.* 2003;9(2):56-61.

29. Harris WS, Gowda M, Kolb JW, Strychacz CP, et al. A randomized, controlled trial of the effects of remote, intercessory prayer on outcomes in patients admitted to the coronary care unit. *Arch Intern Med.* 1999;159:2273-2278.

30. Byrd RC. Positive therapeutic effects of intercessory prayer in a coronary care unit population. *South Med J.* 1988;81:826-829.

31. Cohen K. *The way of qigong: The Art and Science of Chinese Energy Healing.* New York: Ballantine; 1997.

32. Cassel EJ. The nature of suffering and the goals of medicine. *N Engl J Med.* 1982;306(11):639-645.

Chapter Two

Why Spirituality Matters

*Healing and transformation occurs when we deepen
the virtues of faith, love and hope in our lives.*[1]

Christina Puchalski, MD

In the darkness of a winter night in 1986, two people drove along an isolated rural road in northwest New Mexico. Having spent a day hiking, they were returning to the regional medical center in the small town of Gallup, where they both worked. An animal blurred into their path, and the car swerved out of control and flipped over several times before coming to rest.

Thomas Nevola, MD, the driver, perished. His passenger, a colleague from the medical center, survived.

Tom was a senior resident at the Maine-Dartmouth Family Practice Residency, anticipating graduation and beginning practice as a family doctor in June. He was serving a rotation in Pediatrics at Gallup as part of his training.

He was a warm and gregarious man, and his death was a shocking loss to his friends, colleagues and patients back in Maine. Making our way along the process of grief, many of us who knew

Tom began to think about ways that we could honor and celebrate his life, and keep alive his spirit among us.

We recognized that a central theme of Tom's life was his own spirituality, and his efforts to bring his spiritual values and commitments to his work as a doctor. Tom grew up in close-knit working class Roman Catholic family in Rhode Island, and he had always been devoted to his own spiritual journey. Even during 100-hour-a-week clinical rotations, Tom spent some time each day immersed in his collection of spiritual books... I remember the *Confessions of St. Augustine*, in particular... most of which were dog-eared and had bold underlines, stars, arrows and exclamation points page by page.

Arising out of his personal devotions, Tom also spoke freely with his residency and hospital friends about spirituality in medicine. In the month before his death, he set up a grand rounds conference at our affiliated hospital where he invited a number of community clergy to talk with the medical staff about how they might partner together in working with the people whose care they shared; the "patients" at the hospital, the "parishioners" to the clergy. He also joined in some preliminary conversations about developing a chaplaincy program at the hospital, where there had not been one before.

Eventually, the commitment to honor Tom's life led to the inception of an annual symposium, bearing his name, to bring together people from the worlds of health care and spiritual care to talk with one another about healing. The *Tom Nevola, MD Symposium on Spirituality and Health Care* has now been a regular community event for 23 years, and has explored a host of topics in spirituality and health... mental health, addictions, child development, healing and the arts, gratitude, forgiveness, hope, family violence, aging, and love, among others. We usually draw over 200 people, many of whom have returned multiple times.

In the early years of the Nevola Symposium, we presented keynotes and workshops that were heavily weighted toward the issue of why spirituality matters. This was a question, I suppose, that held some lively interest in the late eighties and early nineties. Does the spirituality of our patients really have anything to do with their health? Is this an appropriate topic for health and wellness care? Isn't spirituality a personal and private subject that we should leave to spiritual care professionals to address?

Increasingly, in the years since then, such questions have become less debatable and controversial as the consciousness about spirituality has grown. We have found... particularly for an audience of people who would choose to attend a day-long conference in spirituality and health... that the question of *whether* spirituality matters holds much less interest than the question of *how* spirituality can practically be woven into the process of health and wellness care. Spending too much time on whether, or why, spirituality is important is preaching to the choir. The choir, we have found, is appropriately restless, and wants to move on to practical approaches.

The fact that you are reading these words suggests to me that you are part of the choir. Welcome! I am a charter member of the choir and, in fact, I write this book because I am personally fascinated and compelled by the *practical* issues of how people change and find meaning in their lives. I confess that I am less passionate about the methodological subtleties of the "whether it matters" question than I am passionate about supporting people living their lives with dignity, purpose, direction, and joy. The 47 year old sheet rocker who had a serious back injury and is trying to create a new life. The 55 year old nurse who is trying to make peace with a personal history of severe abuse and to move on. The 32 year old recent immigrant with almost no formal schooling who wants to learn welding so that he can "do a good day's work" and support his young son, whom he cherishes.

Even as I portray myself to you as the practical guy, however, I do also want to share with you some reflections on why spirituality is important in health and wellness care. I think that the context of why spirituality matters can be helpful in laying the groundwork for some of the specific approaches we will be considering.

I want to consider four particular reasons why spirituality is vital to health and wellness care.

SPIRITUALITY IS INTIMATELY RELATED TO HEALTH, WHOLENESS AND WELL-BEING

Historically, spirituality travels together with health and wholeness. Our modern words "health," "whole" and "holy" share a common linguistic ancestor in the Old English word, *"hāl."*

It is certainly my clinical impression over the years that people who have a clear focus on what is "vital and sacred" for them... being a loving partner, being a faithful daughter, being a generous spirit, being someone who can write with incisiveness, being someone who can fix almost anything, being someone who brings calm to chaos... have emotionally richer, more engaged and often healthier lives than people who lack this focus.

As we close in on the end of the first decade of the new century, we can now look back on more than forty years of empirical literature that has explored... and typically supported... these connections. There have been hundreds of credible peer-reviewed studies about spirituality and health; a PubMed search today with the keywords "spirituality" and "health," in fact, yields 2279 citations.

Evolving research in spirituality and health

This literature has been growing exponentially and has been evolving in terms of focus and sophistication. The very early studies of spirituality and health examined health status associated with denominational affiliation. Not surprisingly, religious groups that particularly emphasized nutrition and other healthy lifestyle choices... Mormons, Seventh-Day Adventists, conservative Jews... were found to be healthier overall than the general populations of people who were their peers.

The second wave of research in spirituality-health connections began to explore religious practices. Studies were not just looking at denominational affiliation, but at behavior that was associated with denominational affiliation. Frequent variables that appeared in these studies were religious institution attendance (typically meaning church attendance) and private devotional practices such as Bible-reading, and many of these variables have turned out to be fairly robust predictors of health over the years.

Dr. Harold Koenig, for instance, is a psychiatrist at Duke who is probably the most prolific researcher about spirituality-health connections. In the late 1990s, he and colleagues published several studies of religious activities in older adults, finding that religious service attendance and prayer or Bible study were associated with lower blood pressures (compared with less frequent attenders and study-ers)[2] and that frequent attenders had lower mortality rates than less frequent attenders.[3] In the former study, by the way, people who watched religious TV or listened to religious radio actually had *higher* blood pressures.

The third station in the evolution of this literature has been the increasing emphasis on measures of spirituality, rather than religion. Coincident with the demographic and cultural trends toward a broader expression of spirituality, a number of researchers have developed assessment protocols for research (largely paper-and-pencil) that explore spiritual beliefs and practices that are not necessarily linked to particular religious traditions. Examples in the health literature include INSPIRIT,[4] the SPIRITual history,[5] the Spiritual Involvement and Beliefs Scale,[6] the Functional Assessment of Chronic Illness Therapy- Spiritual Well-Being Scale (FACIT-Sp),[7] and the Spirituality Index of Well-Being.[8] In addition, there are a growing number of clinical protocols and acronyms for spiritual history-taking (largely conversational), notably the FICA questions[9] and the HOPE questions.[10] We will revisit these instruments and issues of spiritual assessment when we consider clinical approaches.

Current research often considers religious and spiritual measures together, with the more personal and individual experience of meaning and purpose inherent in spirituality often showing equivalent and often more substantial associations with health status than measures of religious participation or practice (often referred to as "religiosity"). Daaleman and colleagues, for instance, compared the association of spirituality and religiosity with self-reported health status in geriatric outpatients.[11] Spirituality was measured with the Spirituality Index of Well-Being, which contains items related to self-efficacy (e.g., "There is not much I can do to make a difference in my life") and life scheme (e.g., "I have a lack of purpose in my life"). Religiosity was measured by an aggregate of five questions: frequency of religious service attendance, frequency of private prayer or spiritual practice, self-reported strength of religious or spiritual orientation, closeness to God, and frequency of affective spiritual experiences. Daaleman found that spirituality was related to self-reported health status in this sample, while religiosity was not.

Increasingly, researchers have been exploring dimensions, or components, of spirituality. A particular distinction that has captured a good deal of research attention has been the partitioning of "spiritual well-being" into the methodologically and empirically distinct components of "religious well-being" and "existential well-being." Religious well-being encompasses a variety of religious practices and often pertains to people's perceived relationships with God. Existential well-being pertains to a sense of satisfaction and life purpose. A 2007 study by Tsuang and colleagues, for instance,[12] explored the associations of these two components of spiritual well-being with physical and mental health in 345 pairs of twins from the Vietnam Era Twin Registry. They found that both religious and existential well-being had significant associations with general health and mental health outcomes, but existential well-being had significantly more statistical explanatory power in analyses that controlled for the effects of other variables.

The particular distinction between religious and existential well-being, in fact, appears in a number of current studies. Examples include research that observes more beneficial associations of existential well-being than more specifically religious measures with depression in terminally ill patients in palliative care facilities,[13] with health-related quality of life in cancer survivors,[14] and with suicidality in Croatian war veterans with post-traumatic stress disorder.[15]

Categories of evidence of spirituality-health connections

The proposition that spirituality is related to health, wholeness and well-being is approached in current research in four types of studies; cross-sectional studies with defined populations, longitudinal studies with defined populations, meta-analytic reviews, and intervention studies.

First, *cross-sectional studies* examine spirituality and health variables in defined populations at a single time. Such studies are, by definition, correlational; they may reveal associations but not confirm causality. Some recent examples:

- Finding "strength and comfort from religion," along with participation in social or community groups, had a significant protective effect in mortality rates in patients six months following cardiac surgery.[16]
- Spirituality was strongly associated with life satisfaction and quality of life in prostate cancer and rehabilitation patients.[17]
- Measures of spirituality and spiritual well-being correlated with functional well-being, and test items focused on meaning and peace correlated with physical well-being in women with breast cancer.[18]
- Daily spiritual experiences (such as feeling God's presence, finding comfort in religion and spirituality, being thankful for blessings, feeling selfless caring for others) were associated with decreased alcohol intake, improved quality of life and positive psychosocial status in four multi-ethnic national samples.[19]
- Public religious activity (for men) and both public religious

activity and spiritual experiences were associated with health and well-being in data from the 1998 US General Social Survey.[20]

- Higher measures of spirituality (on the FACIT-Sp) were associated with better health-related quality of life and sexual function in men with prostate cancer.[21]
- Spiritual well-being was significantly related to sleep quality and mental and physical health status in HIV-infected individuals.[22]
- Daily spiritual experiences and not feeling abandoned by God were associated with better emotional health among older male inmates.[23]

Second, *longitudinal studies* examine associations of spirituality and health variables over time. Point-in-time relationships among these variables are fine, but what happens in six weeks? Six months? Two years?

Some clinical issues, where there is a trajectory of effects over time, are particularly suited to prospective longitudinal research. The process of grief after the loss of a loved one is an example of a life experience that typically has a progression over the course of months and, sometimes, years.

Walsh and colleagues looked at the relationship between spirituality and the resolution of bereavement among 135 relatives and close friends of terminally ill patients in a palliative care center in London.[24] They measured spirituality with the Royal Free Interview for religious and spiritual beliefs, which is a well-established scale in visual analogue format that has appeared principally in research in Europe[25] and used a series of core bereavement items to measure intensity of grief. Following patients' deaths, the researchers assessed subjects at 1, 9, and 14 months. They found that subjects with strongly held spiritual beliefs progressed in the resolution of grief across the 14 month study period. Subjects with low strength of belief showed very little change in bereavement at the 9 month point, but recovered by 14 months to a level comparable to the high-belief group. Subjects with no spiritual beliefs, however, showed modest gains in the intensity of grief at the 9 month assessment, but regressed to a renewed intensity of grief seven months later. Their conclusion was that people who hold spiritual beliefs tend to resolve grief more rapidly and completely than people who do not.

Longitudinal studies also examine changes over time with retrospective approaches. Morris, for instance, used a retrospective methodology to study the role of spiritual well-being in the course of coronary artery disease.[26] He was intrigued (as many of us have been) with Dean Ornish's work in reversing coronary artery occlusion with a program of vegetarian diet, regular aerobic exercise and daily meditation, and he hypothesized that Ornish's results would be relatively more or less robust depending on people's spiritual well-being. Morris tracked down the surviving participants in the Lifestyle Heart Trial, which was an intervention program that coached subjects in Ornish's package of lifestyle changes and measured disease progression or regression by catheterization before and after the program. Four years after the conclusion of the Lifestyle Heart Trial, Morris administered Spiritual Orientation Inventories to these surviving subjects, including those who had had the program (an experimental group) and those who had not (a control group).

Morris reported two findings of note. First, he observed that scores on the Spiritual Orientation Inventory correlated significantly with changes in percent stenosis for all of the Lifestyle Heart Trial subjects in both groups. High spirituality scores were associated with the least progression of coronary artery obstruction, and lower scores were associated with the most progression in obstruction. This suggested that something about spiritual well-being, apart from the particulars of the lifestyle intervention program, had a beneficial influence on the progression of coronary disease.

As a comment, I think that this is a remarkable finding. The presumption in mainstream medicine for many years was that "soft" variables like psychological characteristics or psychological approaches had effects on "soft" measures like coping and subjective well-being. In this medical/cultural setting, it would be difficult to find a "harder" variable than coronary artery occlusion. If spirituality has some influence on coronary artery occlusion, this is real science!

Second, Morris found that spirituality measures were substantially higher in people who had been experimental subjects and had participated in the program. This suggested to him that something about the intervention program promoted or fostered the spiritual experience of subjects in the experimental group. It is not hard to speculate that a lifestyle program that emphasized vegetarian diets, self care and meditation in a presumably supportive community setting may have had such effects. This is, of course, why journal articles all conclude with the ritual benediction, "further research is needed." I should learn how to say this in Latin.

It is not uncommon to see such prospective or retrospective longitudinal studies in the literature of spirituality and health. A couple of additional recent examples:

- In a study of 2616 sets of twins from a general population registry, spirituality (religiosity, forgiveness, thankfulness and other such factors) was found to be associated with reduced lifetime risk of "internalizing" (depression, anxiety disorders and eating disorders) and "externalizing" (nicotine dependence, substance abuse and adult antisocial behavior) mental health disorders.[27]
- Using a qualitative research protocol, spiritually based resources (with the over-arching theme of "having an embracing spirit") were found to have beneficial effects on the adaptation of elderly wives of prostate cancer survivors.[28]

A special and most intriguing sub-category of longitudinal spirituality research is the **very-long study**. I suspect I have just coined that term; perhaps, in my long-time adoptive home in Maine, I might have called this type of research the "wicked long study," the adjective "wicked" meaning "IN THE EXTREME." In any case, there are a small number of fascinating spirituality-related research projects that reach across many decades.

Enter the nun study. Beginning in the fall of 1930, young women who were novitiates in a religious order, the American School Sisters of Notre Dame, were asked by the Mother Superior of the order to write autobiographical statements. Many hundreds of young nuns did so, and then went on with their lives and religious careers. Years passed.

Enterprising researchers who had become aware of the existence of these decades-old autobiographical statements in the early 1990s were intrigued to explore the relationship between what these women said sixty years previously with what had become of them in the ensuing time.[29] The researchers contacted sisters who had been born prior to 1917 and obtained permission from 678 of them to allow access to archival data and current health information. Among this group, almost 200 archival autobiographical statements were successfully located. From a research/methodological point of view, women in a religious order make particularly good subjects for longitudinal research because the range of their life experiences… diet, substance use, sexual and relationship history, and so forth… would presumably be narrower than that of the general population; there would be, in other words, fewer potentially confounding variables to consider.

The statements were analyzed and scored with respect to positive emotion and enthusiasm, touching on qualities such as happiness, love, hope, and gratefulness. The low scorers in this analysis tended to have relatively resolute and sterile statements of religious calling, a kind of monotone recitation of; "I am here to do the Lord's work and I will persist through…" The high scorers, in contrast, relatively overflowed with a sense of wonder and joy about the paths upon which they were embarking.

The results were striking. The median age at death among the nuns whose autobiographical expression of positive emotion was in the lowest quartile was 86.6. For nuns whose autobiographical expression of positive emotion was in the highest quartile, the median age at death was 93.5; a difference of 6.9 years. For two other indices of positive emotion, the difference between lowest and highest quartile was even larger. Age at death among nuns who had expressed the largest *number* of positive emotions, for instance, was over ten years greater than nuns who had expressed the lowest number.

Commenting on these data, Martin Seligman points out that the statistical difference between these two groups is greater than the difference that that is typically seen in mortality comparisons between smokers and non-smokers.[30] Most of us in the health professions, appropriately, put considerable emphasis on people's use of tobacco products. The results of this study make me wonder whether, in addition to screening for smoking, we should be screening for joy.

You will note that this research did not analyze the autobiographical statements in terms of "spirituality" in the narrow sense of specifically spiritual or religious language or practices. I would argue, however, that the qualities upon which the nuns were compared… positive emotion, enthusiasm, optimism, passion… tie in very closely with some of the dimensions of spirituality that we have considered. Passionate engagement with life, with the pursuit of values that are "vital and sacred," is deeply spiritual. The word root or "enthusiasm," after all, is "en-theos," which means "God within."

A second wicked long study bears mention, as well. Psychiatrist George Valliant identified Boston-area men in a database dating from before World War II, men from the Harvard classes of 1939-1943 and 456 inner-city contemporaries of these Harvard students.[31] He examined case histories of these people as young men and determined who among them had displayed "mature defenses," which reflected qualities of altruism, humor, future-mindedness and the ability to delay gratification. When surviving men were studied in their elderly years, the men from both groups who had displayed high degrees of mature defenses showed higher income, objective psychosocial adjustment, social supports, marital satisfaction, subjective physical functioning, and joy in living than the men whose ratings of mature defenses had been less.

Another intriguing finding from the Valliant research was that "mature defenses" served to attenuate the effects of severe combat during World War II among the Harvard men. Among the men who had experienced severe combat, the men with the most adaptive defenses showed an average of 0.19 symptoms of Post-traumatic Stress Disorder (PTSD), while the men with the least adaptive defenses showed an average of 1.70 symptoms of PTSD.

The third category of current research about spirituality and health and well-being is the *meta-analytic review.* Rather than reporting original data from single studies, meta-analytic reviews report aggregated data from multiple studies, the rationale being that multiple studies provide perspectives on themes or trends that would be less visible in any single research project.

There have been a number of excellent meta-analytic reviews over the years. The late David Larson, MD, founder of the International Center for the Integration of Health and Spirituality, had a hand in several of these reviews in the 1990s. One such review examined empirical studies that contained at least one measure of religious commitment and at least one measure of physical or mental health status.[32] The data suggested that religious commitment may be beneficial in preventing mental and physical illness, supporting and strengthening people's coping with illness, and facilitating recovery from illness.

A similar review two years later looked specifically at mortality.[33] Larson and colleagues reviewed 42 studies that contained mortality data along with some measure of religiosity. Religiosity was measured in a variety of ways; religious institution attendance, measures of religious coping, measures of private religiousness, measures of religious orientation, and ratings of religion as the greatest source of strength in one's life. Data showed that religious involvement was significantly associated with lower all-cause death rates.

Two meta-analytic reviews, along with very helpful reflections on methodological issues, were included in a sentinel publication in the arena of spirituality and health, the January 2003 issue of *American Psychologist*. In this issue, Powell and colleagues evaluated a number of hypotheses about the linkages of religion and spirituality to physical health.[34] They found that the significantly positive connections were that church attendance protects against death, with some support for the hypotheses that religion or spirituality protects against cardiovascular disease and that being prayed for improves physical recovery from acute illness. Seeman and colleagues looked at evidence for biological pathways connecting religion/spirituality and health, finding support for the linkages of religion/spirituality with cardiovascular, neuroendocrine and immune function.[35]

Since that time, meta-analytic reviews keep coming. Examples include:

- A review of studies of patients with advanced cancer found that psycho-spiritual well-being (self-awareness, coping effectively with stress, connectedness with others, sense of faith, sense of empowerment, and living with meaning and hope) was associated with effective coping with terminal illness and with the ability to find meaning from the experience.[36]
- A review of epidemiological studies of African Americans found that religious participation had a beneficial effect on morbidity/mortality, depressive symptoms, and overall psychological distress.[37]
- A review of 23 studies of spiritual beliefs and practices in patients with cardiac illness (coronary artery bypass graft surgery, congestive heart failure, heart transplants, AMI, blood pressure and healthy-heart promotion) found consistent beneficial effects in the arenas of adaptation and coping... finding comfort, finding meaning, coping, quality

of life, and optimism.[38]

The fourth category of research about spirituality and health and well-being is the *intervention study.* So far, the research that we have reviewed has all been descriptive, exploring relationships that may exist without attempting to influence anything. In contrast to the descriptive approach, there have been a growing number of studies that report on intervention programs... initiatives that attempt to cultivate or to draw upon spiritual resources on behalf of health, healing or well-being. Four recent, substantial examples:

- Working with palliative care patients, Chochinov and Cann developed and evaluated an intervention to enhance the spiritual aspects of dying.[39] "Dignity Therapy" focuses on alleviating depression and suffering, and on supporting patients in finding meaning and purpose. Staff members meet individually with patients to review aspects of life that have been most meaningful for them, the personal history that they most wish to be remembered, and things that need to be said. These sessions are tape recorded, transcribed and returned to the patients "as a tangible product, a legacy, or a generativity document, which in effect allows the patient to leave behind something that will transcend death" (p. S-111). Evaluative results revealed diminished depression and suffering, and enhanced sense of meaning, purpose, dignity and will to live.

- Puchalski and McSkimming chaired an interdisciplinary group that conducted a program on "Creating Healing Environments" at seven medical centers across the country.[40] With some programmatic variation from center to center, the project a) promoted an awareness and cultivation of spirituality in direct caregivers and indirect care providers as a vital aspect of their professional lives, b) supported the development of specific competencies for providing patient-centered spiritual care, and c) developed work-culture interventions that would encourage caregivers to be a consistent and compassionate presence to patients and to one another. A multi-pronged evaluation, surveying patients and staff during the programs and up to one year after the programs had begun, revealed strong positive perceptions of work culture change, greater recognition and support of spiritual issues, and enhanced staff satisfaction.

- Kennedy and colleagues conducted a retreat program for cardiac patients and their partners.[41] In addition to material about healthy lifestyles, the retreats addressed "spiritual principles of healing, including meditation, prayer, forgiveness, and acceptance of what is outside a person's control." Dialogues, as well, challenged participants to find meaning and purpose in their illness. Seventy to ninety percent of the 72 participants reported increased well-being, increased meaning in life, decreased anger, increased connection to others, increased awareness of inner strength and guidance, and increased confidence in handling problems.

- Primary care patients with mood disturbance were given a home study-based spirituality education program.[42] Consisting of eight audio taped teaching sessions, the home study program had a detailed curriculum of spiritual ideas and approaches focused on transcendence, meaning and purpose, connectedness and values. The program was designed to touch on some elements common to different spiritual traditions; "the idea of life's struggles as spiritual teachings," "surrender, forgiveness... unconditional love in challenging circumstances... committing to one's purpose in life... and living in the present" (p.28). Compared with mindfulness meditation and wait-list control groups of the same duration, the spirituality home-study group showed significant enhancements in mood and quality of life.

A category unto itself in the area of intervention studies is the literature on *mindfulness-based approaches*. Popularized and pioneered in America by Dr. Jon Kabat-Zinn, mindfulness consists simply of being aware (or mindful) of present moments, without categorizing, processing or judging. Mindfulness draws energy and attention away from the past and the future, cultivating a rich and non-evaluative experience of present events *externally* (data from the senses like sounds, images, and temperature, and more complicated behavior and interactions of other people) and *internally* (such as somatic sensations, emotions, thoughts and beliefs).

Mindfulness belongs in the conversation about spirituality for three reasons. First, mindfulness has its origins in Eastern (particularly, Buddhist) spiritual traditions and overlaps substantially with contemplative practices in a variety of spiritual traditions world-wide. Second, the notion of non-judgmental perception of present moments overlaps with spiritual ideas and practices of non-attachment, transcendence, and gratefulness. And third, mindful awareness in practice is often paired with emphasis on intentional living in faithfulness to personally meaningful values.

Kabat-Zinn and colleagues and students have focused mindfulness approaches into programs of mindfulness-based stress reduction (MBSR) that have been offered internationally for many years. MBSR teaches skills of compassionate awareness and presence (what Shapiro[43] calls "kind, open acceptance of all experiences") typically in group settings over a number of weeks. A sampling of outcomes of MBSR programs from the last three or four years:

- Reductions in perceived stress, depression and pain, increased mindfulness and energy in a community sample.[44]
- Improvement in quality of life, joy in life, tension, physical symptoms, anger, and vigor in oncology patients.[45]
- Enhanced quality of life, decreased stress symptoms, and beneficially altered cortisol and immune patterns in subjects with breast and with prostate cancer.[46]
- Improvements in burnout symptoms, relaxation, and life satisfaction among nurses and nurse aides.[47]

- Immediate and three-year follow-up improvement in pain, quality of life, coping with pain, anxiety, depression and somatic complaints among female patients with fibromyalgia.[48]
- Reduced cortisol levels, increased quality of life, and increased coping effectiveness in early stage breast cancer patients.[49]
- Improved psychological distress and strengthened well-being in patients with rheumatoid arthritis.[50]

And a couple of recent meta-analyses for good measure:

- Favorable changes in quality of life, coping styles, mood disturbance, and adjustment to cancer in seven methodologically-appropriate studies of patients with cancer.[51]
- Improvements in mood, sleep quality and reductions in stress in ten qualifying studies in cancer care in the UK.[52]

So... **what is going on here?**

Amidst the large literature about spirituality and health, there have been a modest number of scientists who have made serious attempts to develop comprehensive models about *why* there should be such associations. If spirituality does indeed influence health and wellness, how does this happen?

No one has explored such questions in a more substantial and articulate way than Jeff Levin. A social epidemiologist and gerontologist, Dr. Levin was a faculty member at the Department of Family and Community Medicine at Eastern Virginia Medical School until he left the academic world to become a philosopher-farmer-writer in rural Kansas in the late 1990s. He published some of the sentinel articles in the epidemiology of religion and health during his formal academic career[53-56] and has continued to address and develop these subjects in peer-reviewed journals[57] and books[58] in his current life as an independent researcher and consultant.

Levin proposes that there are five pathways that could mediate the associations between spirituality and health status.[57] First, there is good evidence, he argues, for **biological** pathways. He points to data on disease incidence in defined religious groups (lower cancer rates in Hutterites, higher rates of familial hypercholesterolemia in Dutch Reformed Afrikaaners) and suggests that the insular nature of these communities keeps them biologically distinct, thus maintaining genetic or hereditary factors that relate to health.

Second, he points to a variety of **psychosocial** pathways that follow from religious and spiritual involvement, such as health-related behaviors, social support, positive emotions, beneficial health beliefs and personality styles, and positive thoughts. Such mechanisms, he argues, may be applicable both in the primary prevention of illnesses and in the effectiveness of spiritual interventions like prayer, laying-on-of-hands and spiritual healing.

Third, Levin suggests that spirituality and health associations may be mediated by **bioenergy-based** pathways. Most world cultures and spiritual traditions, dating from thousands of years ago, have had beliefs about vital life forces… such as *qi* or *prana*… that are central to wellness and that may be focused or directed in spiritual healing. The phrase, "subtle energies" is often used in modern consideration of bioenergy-based systems and effects. There have been some efforts to measure these forces, but they remain largely hypothetical, with the literature predominantly addressing health effects of interventions (such as Ayurveda or traditional Chinese medicine) presumed to operate by means of such forces.

Fourth, Levin says that there may be **nonlocal** pathways. "Nonlocal" effects would operate in ways that are independent of space and time. The beneficial effects of distant intercessory prayer in a landmark study with a coronary care unit population, for instance,[59] would not be explained by biological, psychosocial or local/bioenergy mechanisms, since there was no contact between pray-ers and prayed-for patients, nor were patients aware that they were being prayed for.

Finally, there is the possibility of **supernatural** pathways. It is conceivable, Levin says, that healing effects may be associated with the volitional action of a Divine being or force, operating outside of the natural universe. This is, he says, not testable or knowable… you can't use naturalistic methodologies to evaluate something outside of the realm of the natural world… but the fact that this is not knowable does not mean that it does not exist.

SPIRITUALITY MEDIATES CHOICES IN HEALTH BEHAVIORS

Why *should* someone stop smoking, anyway? If you are diabetic, why *should* you care what your A1c is?

It seems to me that *health* really does not have much inherent value for anybody; it matters only insofar as it is instrumental in enabling us to live our lives in ways that are meaningful for us. In an earlier incarnation as a substance abuse counselor, I concluded that most of the addicts I worked with really didn't care much about abstinence/sobriety per se, but made changes because abstinence/sobriety was linked to what was "vital and sacred" for them… maintaining a relationship with a loved one, taking pride in standing on one's own two feet, or being the kind of person that a young son could look up to. Stopping smoking, similarly, is usually important not for some amorphous health reasons, but because someone would be able to be a better example to a child, to play with a grandchild, to work in the garden and grow flowers next summer, to put food on the table, or to walk in the woods in the fall.

Psychologist David Waters PhD from the University of Virginia makes similar assumptions and has developed a framework in which he emphasizes the relationship of "health goals" and "life goals." "Health goals" are the choices and lifestyle behaviors that people can pursue in order to address their most important health issues. Exercising, stopping smoking, developing a good nutritional plan. "Life goals" touch on the things that are most important to people in their lives… the things that they care about the most. Being a better teacher, coaching young people, being able to work in stained glass.

Speaking at a national meeting of the Society of Teachers of Family Medicine in 2006, Waters proposed that doctors often presume that patients will be invested in health goals without understanding patients' life goals, resulting in mutual frustration and thwarting progress toward patients' health and wellness. He argues that it is essential for doctors… and, by inference, all of us as providers of health and wellness care… to first understand patients' life values, then to present a menu of choices in health goals that would potentially serve the life goals that patients are identifying. The formula is "What is really important in my life is _____; therefore, my health goals are _____."

A recent patient is active in Buddhist practices and wishes to stop smoking. She comments,

"Health" is not enough to motivate me to stop smoking. My reasons for stopping need to be more important than my reasons to smoke. I have taken a vow to work toward enlightenment, for me, and to help other people toward enlightenment. Smoking obstructs the inner channels where the chakras are… if I am serious about enlightenment, I have to quit.

One of my favorite observations about change comes from organizational consultant Margaret Wheatley. "Real change," she says, "comes from the simple act of people talking about what they care about."[60] Focusing on people's life goals…what they really care about…creates energy and motivation that can prompt "real change."

You will see, in the preceding paragraphs, the connection with spirituality. Spirituality as what is "vital and sacred," what is ultimately and deeply important to people, meshes smoothly with Waters' idea of "life goals" and with Wheatley's idea of "what [people] care about."

SPIRITUALITY OFTEN FRAMES THE WAYS THAT PEOPLE COPE WITH ADVERSITY AND PURSUE THE JOURNEY TOWARD WELLNESS/WHOLENESS

We have reviewed a number of examples of the substantial literature on spirituality and health, which has a lot to say about spiritually-based coping, well-being and quality of life. Let's approach this in more of a clinical way.

> *I have a 47 year old patient with recurrent ovarian cancer. She has had an off and on relationship with a husband who I think has been abusing prescription drugs… he is not my patient… and is often the single parent of daughters in their teens. She has lots of reasons to be overwhelmed and angry, but she is usually among the most cheerful and optimistic people I see. When I pointed this out to her a year or so ago, she said that she turns it all over to God, and that God sets her on the right path. I'm not sure whether this will heal her cancer, but she certainly has had some healing in how she lives her life.*

The story from this primary care physician is not unusual. Even in my part of the world, the Laconic New Englander Belt, if you ask most people what sustains them through hard times or what energizes them in the journey toward wholeness, they will typically make reference to spiritual values or a spiritual presence… "God," "my spirituality," "the Man Upstairs," "being there for my children," and so forth.

As I speak with people about coping and wholeness, I hear regular examples of each of the five dimensions of spirituality that we reviewed in the last chapter. People turn to spiritual community. They find renewal and comfort in spiritually-based practices and rituals. They are sustained as they find meaning and purpose in their life experience. (You may recall the famous assertion of Viktor Frankl, concentration camp survivor, psychiatrist, author of *Man's Search for Meaning,* that "Those who have a *why* to live, can bear with almost any *how*.") People are energized by engaging their passions. And frequently, people find strength and direction in their relationships with a divine presence.

In other words, people do frequently draw upon spiritual values, practices and relationships for support and direction. Given that these values and resources matter to people and make a difference in their journeys of coping and wholeness, it is important for us to understand and to help patients nurture these values and practices as much as we can.

SPIRITUALITY IS IMPORTANT BECAUSE PEOPLE WANT TO BE KNOWN IN THIS WAY BY THEIR CAREGIVERS

We have considered the importance of spirituality in health and wellness care because of associations of spirituality with health status and well-being, because spiritual values energize health behavior choices, and because spirituality is often a wellspring of strength and direction in the journey toward coping and wholeness. The final reason why spirituality matters in health and wellness care is because patients *want it to be* part of health and wellness care. Patients want to be known in this way by their caregivers.

A patient tells me, "You seem to really want to know who I am and what I want for my life… you seem to really believe in me… that is so important to me." I hear comments like this frequently from physicians and from patients about their physicians.

I saw a 19 year old young woman for a urinary tract infection. Asking about sexual practices, she admitted that she had had unprotected sex with a series of one-time partners in the past few months, one resulting in a pregnancy and miscarriage. She was sad and teary telling me this story, the background being that she had been marginalized and maybe abused by her family growing up and had moved out on her own when she dropped out of school in the 11th grade. I asked her what she wanted for her life and she said that she always wanted to be a teacher. Why did she want this… because she thought she could

*really make a difference with kids who grew up as lost as she had been.
We dealt with the UTI, but we spent more time talking about her
being a bright young woman who really could begin to put together the
wonderful dreams that she had for her life, starting with making some
better choices about her relationships with men. When she left, she said
how much she appreciated my taking the time to get to know her and
some of the things that were important to her.*

As we have discussed before, this story from a family physician is not about "religion," and may not have specifically involved spiritual language. It is, however, a wonderful example of
good spiritual care in the broad sense of looking with patients at
"the vital and sacred," the things in patients' lives that give them
meaning and energy.

There have been a number of studies in the medical literature
about patients' interests in incorporating spirituality in their health
care. McCord and a small army of colleagues (14 co-authors…
one can picture animated discussions around the table) surveyed
almost a thousand patients in medical practices in Ohio about
their perspectives on physician discussions of spirituality.[61] They
found that eighty three percent of respondents wanted physicians
to ask about spiritual beliefs in at least some circumstances. The
most frequently identified circumstances were life threatening illnesses (77%), serious medical conditions (74%) and loss of loved
ones (70%). Overwhelmingly, the patients who were interested in
discussions of spirituality indicated that such discussions would increase physician-patient understanding, helping physicians to encourage realistic hope, give focused medical advice, and sometimes
change medical treatment.

Very recently, Scott and colleagues explored the meaning of
healing relationships in primary care.[62] Using a qualitative methodology, they interviewed a small number of primary care clinicians
who had been identified as exemplary healers, along with patients of
those physicians with whom the physicians judged they had healing

relationships. In the content analysis of interview data, a number of processes were identified that foster healing relationships, having to do with non-judgment, collaboration and commitment. The results of these processes... the relational outcomes that patients valued... were trust, hope and being known. Speaking of being known, the authors quote a patient commenting how important it is to her to have a physician who "knows who I am first of all... knows exactly who I am."

When we know where people are in the broad areas of human experience subsumed by spirituality... spiritual community, spiritual practices, meaning and purpose, passions, and relationships with spirit... we know them deeply. This makes for healing relationships and underscores the importance of incorporating spirituality in whole-person health and wellness care.

SUMMARY

We have considered four reasons why spirituality matters in health and wellness care.

- Spirituality is intimately related to health, wholeness and well-being.
  - o Research about spirituality and health has exploded in quantity and substantially advanced in sophistication in the last twenty years.
  - o Categories of empirical evidence about spirituality-health connections include:
    - Cross-sectional studies (examining spirituality and health variables in defined populations at a single time)
    - Longitudinal studies (examining associations of spirituality and health variables over time). The *wicked-long* study is a subcategory here.
    - Meta-analytic reviews (reporting aggregated data from multiple studies)

- Intervention studies (reporting results of intervention projects that attempt to cultivate or to draw upon spiritual resources on behalf of health, healing or well-being). Research on mindfulness-based approaches merits particular mention here.
  - A particularly articulate synthesis of potential mechanisms of spirituality-health associations comes from epidemiologist Jeff Levin, who proposes five possible pathways:
    - Biological
    - Psychosocial
    - Bioenergy-based
    - Nonlocal
    - Supernatural
- Spirituality mediates choices in health behaviors.
- Spirituality often frames the ways that people cope with adversity and pursue the journey toward wellness/wholeness.
- Spirituality is important because people want to be known in this way by their caregivers.

REFERENCES

1. Puchalski C. Forgiveness: Spiritual and medical implications. *The Yale Journal for Humanities in Medicine.* September 18 2002.
2. Koenig HG, George LK, Hays JC, Larson DB, Cohen HJ, Blazer DG. The relationship between religious activities and blood pressure in older adults. *Int J Psychiatry Med.* 1998;28(2):189-213.
3. Koenig HG, Hays JC, Larson DB, et al. Does religious attendance prolong survival? A six-year follow-up study of 3,968 older adults. *J Gerontol A Biol Sci Med Sci.* Jul 1999;54(7):M370-376.
4. VandeCreek L, Ayres S, Bassham M. Using INSPIRIT to conduct spiritual assessments. *J Pastoral Care.* Spring 1995;49(1):83-89.
5. Maugans TA. The SPIRITual history. *Arch Fam Med.* Jan 1996;5(1):11-16.
6. Hatch RL, Burg MA, Naberhaus DS, Hellmich LK. The Spiritual Involvement and Beliefs Scale. Development and testing of a new instrument. *J Fam Pract.* Jun 1998;46(6):476-486.

7. Peterman AH, Fitchett G, Brady MJ, Hernandez L, Cella D. Measuring spiritual well-being in people with cancer: The Functional Assessment of Chronic Illness Therapy- Spiritual Well-Being Scale (FACIT-Sp). *Annals of Beh Med.* 2002;24(1):49-58.

8. Daaleman T, Frey B. The spirituality index of well-being: A new instrument for health-related quality-of-life research. *Arch Fam Med.* 2004;2:499-503.

9. Puchalski CM. Taking a spiritual history: FICA. *Spirituality and medicine connection.* 1999;3(1):1.

10. Anandarajah G, Hight E. Spirituality and medical practice: using the HOPE questions as a practical tool for spiritual assessment. *Am Fam Physician.* Jan 1 2001;63(1):81-89.

11. Daaleman T, Perera S, Studenski S. Religion, spirituality and health status in geriatric outpatients. *Annals of Fam Med.* 2004;2(1):49-53.

12. Tsuang MT, Simpson JC, Koenen KC, Kremen WS, Lyons MJ. Spiritual well-being and health. *J Nerv Mental Dis.* 2007;195(8):673-680.

13. Nelson CJ, Rosenfeld B, Breitbart W, Galietta M. Spirituality, religion, and depression in the terminally ill. *Psychosomatics.* 2002;43(3):213-220.

14. Edmondson D, Park CL, Blank TO, Fenster JR, Mills MA. Deconstructing spiritual well-being: existential well-being and HRQOL in cancer survivors. *Psycho-Oncology.* 2008;17:161-169.

15. Nad S, Marcinko D, Vuksan-Aeusa B, Jakovljevic M, Jakovljevic G. Spiritual well-being, intrinsic religiosity, and suicidal behavior in predominantly Catholic Croatian war veterans with chronic post-traumatic stress disorder: A case control study. *J Nerv Mental Dis.* 2008;196(1):79-83.

16. Oxman TE, Freeman DH, Jr., Manheimer ED. Lack of social participation or religious strength and comfort as risk factors for death after cardiac surgery in the elderly. *Psychosom Med.* Jan-Feb 1995;57(1):5-15.

17. Tate D, Forcheimer M. Quality of life, life satisfaction, and spirituality: Comparing outcomes between rehabilitation and cancer patients. *Am J Phys Med Rehabil.* 2002;81(6):400-410.

18. Levine E, Targ E. Spiritual correlates of functional well-being in women with breast cancer. *Integr Cancer Ther.* 2002;1(2):166-174.

19. Underwood L, Terisi J. The daily spiritual experience scale: development, theoretical description, reliability, exploratory factor analysis, and preliminary construct validity using health-related data. *Annals of Beh Med.* 2002;24(1):22-33.

20. Maselko J, Kubzansky L. Gender differences in religious practices, spiritual experiences and health: Results from the US General Social Survey. *Soc Sci Med.* 2002;62(11):2848-2860.

21. Krupski T, Kwan L, Fink A, Sonn G, Maliski S, Litwin M. Spirituality influences health related quality of life in men with prostate cancer. *Psycho-Oncology.* 2006;15:121-131.

22. Phillips K, Mock K, Bopp C, Dudgeon W, Hand GA. Spiritual well-being, sleep disturbance, and mental and physical health status in HIV-infected individuals. *Issues in Mental Health Nursing.* 2006;27:125-139.

23. Allen R, Phillips L, Roff L, Cavanaugh R, Day L. Religiousness/spirituality and mental health among older male inmates. *Gerontologist.* 2008;48(5):692-697.

24. Walsh K, King M, Jones L, Tookman A, Blizard R. Spiritual beliefs may affect outcome of bereavement: Prospective study. *BMJ.* 2002;324(7353):1551.

25. King M, Speck P, Thomas A. The Royal Free interview for religious and spiritual beliefs: Development and standardization. *Psychol Med.* 1995;25(6):1125-1134.

26. Morris E. The relationship of spirituality to coronary heart disease. *Alt Therapies.* 2001;7(5):96-98.

27. Kendler K, Liu X, Gardner C, McCullough M, Larson D, Prescott C. Dimensions of religiosity and their relationship to lifetime psychiatric and substance use disorders. *Am J Psychiatry.* 2003;160(3):496-503.

28. Ka'opua L, Gotay C, Boehm P. Spiritually based resources in adaptation to long-term prostate cancer survival: Perspectives of elderly wives. *Health and Soc Work.* 2007;32(1):29-39.

29. Danner D, Snowdon D, Friesen W. Positive emotions in early life and longevity: Findings from the nun study. *J Pers Soc Psych.* 2001;80(5):804-813.

30. Seligman M. *Authentic Happiness.* New York: Free Press; 2002.

31. Vaillant G. Adaptive mental mechanisms: Their role in a positive psychology. *Am Psychologist.* 2000;55(1):89-98.

32. Matthews DA, McCullough ME, Larson DB, Koenig HG, Swyers JP, Milano MG. Religious commitment and health status: A review of the research and implications for family medicine. *Arch Fam Med.* Mar-Apr 1998;7(2):118-124.

33. McCullough ME, Hoyt WT, Larson DB, Koenig HG, Thoresen C. Religious involvement and mortality: A meta-analytic review. *Health Psychol.* May 2000;19(3):211-222.

34. Powell LH, Shahabi L, Thoresen C. Religion and spirituality: Linkages to physical health. *Am Psychologist.* 2003;58(1):36-52.

35. Seeman TE, Dubin LF, Seeman M. Religion/spirituality and health: A critical review of the evidence for biological pathways. *Am Psychologist.* 2003;58(1):53-63.

36. Lin H, Bauer-Wu S. Psycho-spiritual well-being in patients with advanced cancer: An integrative review of the literature. *J Adv Nursing.* 2003;44(1):69-80.

37. Levin J, Chatters L, Taylor R. Religion, health and medicine in African Americans: Implications for physicians. *J Natl Med Assoc.* 2005;97(2):237-249.

38. Villagomeza L. Mending broken hearts: The role of spirituality in cardiac illness: a research synthesis, 1991-2004. *Holist Nurs Pract.* 2006;20(4):169-186.

39. Chochinov H, Cann B. Interventions to enhance the spiritual aspects of dying. *J Palliat Med.* 2005;8 Suppl 1:S103-115.

40. Puchalski CM, McSkimming S. Creating healing environments: An initiative seeks to restore "heart and humanity" to depersonalized health care. *Health Progress.* 2006;87(3).

41. Kennedy J, Abbott R, Rosenberg B. Changes in spirituality and well-being in a retreat program for cardiac patients. *Altern Ther Health Med.* 2002;8(4):64-73.

42. Moritz S, Quan H, Rickhi B, et al. A home study-based spirituality education program decreases emotional distress and increases quality of life--a randomized, controlled trial. *Altern Ther Health Med.* 2006;12(6):26-35.

43. Shapiro S, Carlson L, Astin J, Freedman B. Mechanisms of mindfulness. *J Clin Psychol.* 2006;62(3):373-386.

44. Smith B, Shelley B, Dalen J, Wiggins K, Tooley E, Bernard J. A pilot study comparing the effects of mindfulness-based and cognitive-behavioral stress reduction. *J Alt Comp Med.* 2008;14(3):251-258.

45. Kieviet-Stijnen A, Visser A, Garssen B, Hudig W. Mindfulness-based stress reduction training for oncology patients: Patients' appraisal and changes in well-being. *Pt Educ Couns.* 2008;72(3):436-442.

46. Carlson L, Speca M, Faris P, Patel K. One year pre-post intervention follow-up of psychological, immune, endocrine and blood pressure outcomes of mindfulness-based stress reduction (MBSR) in breast and prostate cancer outpatients. *Brain Beh Immun.* 2007;21(8):1038-1049.

47. Mackenzie C, Poulin P, Seidman-Carlson R. A brief mindfulness-based stress reduction intervention for nurses and nurse aides. *Appl Nurs Res.* 2006;19(2):105-109.

48. Grossman P, Tiefenthaler-Gilmer U, Raysz A, Kesper U. Mindfulness training as an intervention for fibromyalgia: Evidence of postintervention and 3-year follow-up benefits in well-being. *Psychother Psychosom.* 2007;76(4):226-233.

49. Witek-Janusek L, Albuquerque K, Chroniak K, Chroniak C, Durazo-Arvizu R, Mathews H. Effect of mindfulness based stress reduction on immune function, quality of life and coping in women newly diagnosed with early stage breast cancer. *Brain Beh Immun.* 2008;22(6):969-981.

50. Pradhan E, Baumgarten M, Langenberg P, et al. Effect of Mindfulness-Based Stress Reduction in rheumatoid arthritis patients. *Arthritis Rheum.* 2007;57(7):1116-1118.

51. Matchim Y, Armer J. Measuring the psychological impact of mindfulness meditation on health among patients with cancer: A literature review. *Oncol Nurs Forum.* 2007;34(5):1059-1066.

52. Smith J, Richardson J, Hoffman C, Pilkington K. Mindfulness-based stress reduction as supportive therapy in cancer care: Systematic review. *J Adv Nursing.* 2005;52(3):315-327.

53. Levin J, Vanderpool HY. Is religion therapeutically significant for hypertension? *Soc Sci Med.* 1989;29(1):67-78.

54. Levin JS. Religion and health: Is there an association, is it valid, and is it causal? *Soc Sci Med.* Jun 1994;38(11):1475-1482.

55. Levin JS. How prayer heals: A theoretical model. *Altern Ther Health Med.* Jan 1996;2(1):66-73.

56. Levin JS. How religion influences morbidity and health: Reflections on natural history, salutogenesis and host resistance. *Soc Sci Med.* Sep 1996;43(5):849-864.

57. Levin J. Spiritual determinants of health and healing: An epidemiologic perspective on salutogenic mechanisms. *Alt Therapies.* 2003;9(6):48-57.

58. Levin J. *God, Faith and Health: Exploring the Spirituality-Healing Connection.* New York: Wiley; 2001.

59. Bryd R. Positive therapeutic effects of intercessory prayer in a coronary care unit population. *Southern Med J.* 1988;81:826-829.

60. Wheatley M. *Turning to One Another: Simple Conversations to Restore Hope to the Future.* San Francisco: Berrett-Koehler; 2002.

61. McCord G, Gilchrist V, Grossman S, et al. Discussing spirituality with patients: A rational and ethical approach. *Ann Fam Med.* 2004;2(4):356-361.

62. Scott J, Cohen D, Dicicco-Bloom B, Miller W, Stange K, Crabtree B. Understanding healing relationships in primary care. *Ann Fam Med.* 2008;6(4).

Chapter Three

Who Provides Spiritual Care?

*Everybody can be great... because anybody can serve. You don't have
to have a college degree to serve. You don't have to
make your subject and verb agree to serve.
You only need a heart full of grace, a soul generated by love.*

Martin Luther King, Jr.

In front of you is the diabetic woman who weighs 340 pounds and
has serious leg ulcers. Or the young mother who is overwhelmed and
demoralized with two infant children and an inattentive partner.
Or the previously tireless Little League coach who was disabled in
an industrial accident. Or the teenager who has been smoking cigarettes for three years, with considerable mixed feelings. Or the man
with the chronic cough and suspicious shadow on the lung X-ray.

Who cares for these people? Who partners with you in caring
for these people? What does it mean to provide *spiritual* care to
these and the limitless variety of other people whom you see in
your professional work?

It is generally assumed that spiritual care is provided by spiritual
care professionals. The June 2006 issue of the *Southern Medical*

Journal, for instance, featured a series of articles (arising out of that journal's "Spirituality/Medicine Interface Project") highlighting the contribution of pastoral care professionals to the healing process.[1] Describing chaplains as "hidden assets," the introduction to this special section emphasized the specific training, knowledge, and expertise of chaplains, noting, however, that it was "not our intention to advocate that clinicians attend to the spiritual needs of patients under their care."

There is, of course, a sense in which this perspective is true. Our spiritual care colleagues... chaplains, clergy, spiritual directors... are the experts in spiritual care. They typically have had theological education and often have had specialized clinical training in clinical pastoral education ("CPE"), which is the nationally-systematized clinical training program for spiritual caregivers. Our spiritual care colleagues spend substantial time with patients and families and are skilled with a range of approaches... spiritual assessment techniques, taxonomies of spiritual issues and needs, devotional practices, and relationships with sacred texts, among many others... for understanding and healing the spiritual woundedness of people.

But the expertise of spiritual care professionals does not diminish the ways in which health and wellness care clinicians play vital roles in spiritual care. After all, the expertise of tertiary care cardiologists does not diminish the role that primary care physicians, naturopaths, behavioral health consultants, and nutritionists play in addressing cardiac disease. The question is... what is the role of those of us who are not spiritual care specialists, and how do we collaborate with our spiritual care colleagues in the larger picture of providing spiritual care?

PATIENT AND CLINICIAN PERSPECTIVES ON SPIRITUAL CARE

Daaleman and colleagues reported a qualitative investigation that speaks to this question.[2] Working in a palliative care setting, they explored the perceptions of spiritual care held by patients and health care providers. Their approach was to invite dying patients and their family members to identify clinicians and other health care workers who had provided spiritual care at the end of life, to "identify specific individuals who were most involved in the patients' spiritual care." A total of 38 patients and 65 family members identified 237 spiritual caregivers; 95 (41%) family or friends, 38 (17%) clergy, and 66 (29%) clinicians and other health care workers. A second stage sampling procedure resulted in the identification of 12 spiritual caregivers identified by dying patients and their family members for detailed study. Among the final 12 study subjects, 8 were physicians, 2 were chaplains/pastoral caregivers, 1 was a nurse and 1 worked in facilities services/housekeeping.

Interviews with these 12 study participants revealed three major themes as core elements of spiritual care in this setting. The core elements were

- "Being present" (intentionality in attention to emotional, social and spiritual needs),
- "Opening eyes" (patient and caregiver recognizing the human dimension in one another), and
- "Co-creating" (collaboration in developing holistic care plans that would maintain the humanity and dignity of patients in the face of death).

Daaleman noted the "marked absence of explicitly religious practices or beliefs in our data," commenting that "our participants reported that spiritual care was provided to individuals who were present to them in the context of recognized human value, dignity and shared decision-making, rather than through shared practices (i.e., prayer) or through discussions of religious or theological issues at the bedside," and that "our framework suggests that spiritual care may be effectively and interchangeably provided by multiple members of the care team" (p. 410).

I find this a very encouraging summary. Daaleman's findings... grounded in the perspectives and experience of patients, families and health care workers… highlight "being present," "dignity and shared decision-making," and "multiple members of the health care team." A good template; being present to people, helping people to make choices arising from their values, and members of health care teams working together. While not diminishing the role of specialist spiritual caregivers, it points to three substantial roles in spiritual care for those if us who are providers of health and wellness care.

CONTRIBUTIONS TO SPIRITUAL CARE BY PROVIDERS OF HEALTH AND WELLNESS CARE

As we consider the roles that those of us who are clinicians play in spiritual care, we should begin with a working definition of spiritual care. A perspective that particularly resonates with me comes from palliative care and hospice consultant J. S. Lunn;

"Meeting people where they are and assisting them in connecting or reconnecting to things, practices, ideas, and principles that are at their core of their being… the breath of their life, making a connection between yourself and that person."[3]

You will note the close relationship of this perspective with Koop's view of spirituality as "the vital center of a person, that which is held sacred." We might, in fact, truncate the Lunn definition to the idea of "assisting people to connect with what is "vital and sacred" in their lives." Or, simpler still (I have always thought that we deserve extra credit for using common-English words):

Helping people to connect with the things that really matter to them.

I believe that clinicians… and, for that matter, non-clinical members of health care teams, as Daaleman found… contribute to this vision of spiritual care in three ways.

Intention and presence

First, we come to people with compassionate, healing intention and with genuine presence.

I have a 56 year old female patient with a long list of medical problems... hypertension, diabetes, fibromyalgia, depression... that were really daunting when I first met her. She was pretty tentative with me at first. We tinkered with antihypertension meds and talked about her diabetic care. As we got to know one another, she slowly began to tell me some stories about her life. She had grown up in a reasonably happy family but always felt driven to excel. I think she really put a lot of pressure on herself... in school and in music mostly, and apparently did quite well although it was stressful for her. She married young but could never have children, which I gradually recognized was a great sadness in her life. Her husband took up with another woman and she has been alone... and lonely... for several years. At her low point, her hypertension and diabetes weren't under very good control and she had dropped away from playing music in the community. As she told me some of these stories, I noticed more of a spark in her every time I saw her. I think I came to the conclusion that my relationship with her was not so much about prescribing meds as it was about creating a safe place where she knew that somebody would care about and honor her journey... and maybe give her the chance to sort some things out by talking. Interestingly, over the months, she lost some weight and got her hypertension and diabetes back under good control.

The importance of intention and presence in spiritual care cannot be underestimated. I hear stories of intention and presence consistently as I talk with health and wellness care clinicians about the times when they feel that they have really connected with patients in meaningful ways. The keywords often are "caring," "just listening," "honoring," "felt privileged," "safe place," "sacred," "touched," and so forth. In the language of logic (remember this from high school math?), I think that intention and presence are "necessary" and often "sufficient" in spiritual care.

The foundational role of intention and presence in spiritual care is frequently described in the health care literature, as well. Christina Puchalski, MD, geriatric physician and founder of the George Washington Institute for Spirituality and Health, speaks of "fully present care"[4] and "compassionate care."[5] She makes the point (which we will explore further) that compassionate care is important not only because it allows caregivers to be fully present and supportive to patients, but also because it sets the stage for caregivers to be open to their own intuition in understanding and caring for patients. Puchalski also makes the distinction between "intrinsic" aspects of spiritual care (compassionate and altruistic care giving) and "extrinsic" elements of spiritual care (spiritual history-taking, assessment of spiritual issues and resources, and incorporation of patients' spiritual beliefs and practices into plans of care).

Similarly, Gowri Anandarajah, MD, Director of the family medicine residency at Brown and frequent author in the field, draws a distinction between "specialized" and "general" spiritual care.[6] Specialized spiritual care, she argues, is typically the domain of spiritual care professionals, while general spiritual care... compassion, presence, true listening, and the encouragement of realistic hope... pertain to all of us as clinicians. "These elements," she comments, "do not require doing, but rather being. These interventions do not require inquiring about specific beliefs and require no more time than a clinician's usual duties. Rather, they require that health care professionals augment their everyday activities with presence, compassion and positive intention" (p. 452)

The case for intention and presence, I hope, is affirming to providers of health and wellness care. To audiences of people like the physician at the beginning of the Introduction, who are apprehensive about potentially daunting theological overtones of "spiritual care," I emphasize that *you do this already*. You know how to do this. This arises out of who you are as a healer. And, typically, you do this well.

We will explore further the reasons why intention and presence matter, and give substantial attention to how intention and presence are cultivated, in Chapter 7.

Positive spirituality, issues and resources

The spirit with which we come to people is the foundation of spiritual care, but there is more. Not only does our intention and presence as clinicians matter, but the conversation matters, as well.

I have written elsewhere about the distinction between spiritual issues and spiritual resources.[7] Suffering, particularly in the setting of serious illness, disability and loss, often involves spiritual issues. What do you say to a 29 year old mother of two infant children who has just been diagnosed with end-stage breast cancer, whose view of the world as a safe and gentle place has been completely shattered? What do you say to parents of a beautiful young child who has been disfigured in a fire… who are absolutely furious at God for allowing such egregious suffering? What do you say to the aging man who feels estranged from his faith and is increasingly despondent that he may never be able to heal a decades-long rift with his son?

These are spiritual issues… points of suffering that call into question people's fundamental beliefs about themselves and the universe and how it all fits together. Typically, the healing of spiritual issues is the job of spiritual care specialists.

Spiritual resources, however, are different. All of us who provide health and wellness care can be attentive to and nurture the values, beliefs and practices that sustain and empower people.

Bob had been sober for two years, but he was teetering. Financial problems, painful breakup with his fiancée… he was demoralized and had a lot of doubts about whether he could make it. I asked him if he had gone through hard times like this before. Not to this extent, he said, but a number of times he could remember when he lay awake worrying about the struggles in his life. What kept him going during these times?

He paused. "I guess what comes to mind," he said, "is the idea that 'to get out of your head, go help somebody else.'" He came back the next week feeling more optimistic… he had taken a more active role in a couple of 12-step meetings and had spent some considerable time with a young man who was new to the program, to get him going. This didn't fix his money problems or heal the hurt of the breakup, he emphasized, but it reminded him that he was "bigger than these problems."

For Bob, "getting out of your head by helping somebody else" is an important spiritual value; it forms part of what is "vital and sacred" in his life. When he is giving expression to this value, his energy is very different from what it is when he is not. The caregiver, a social worker, provides good spiritual care by drawing attention to this valued resource and inviting Bob to again make this a part of his life. The story is a good example of our definition of spiritual care; "helping people to connect with the things that really matter to them."

All of us provide spiritual care by exploring with people a host of similar questions oriented to spiritual resources and "positive spirituality."

- *"What are the things that are really important to you?"*
- *"What do you take pride in?"*
- *"What do you hope for?"*
- *"Where do you find strength… what sustains you… what helps you to keep going?"*
- *"What helps you to be more peaceful and centered?"*
- *"What do you hope the legacy of your life will be?"*
- *"What are you really passionate about?"*
- *"When do you feel most alive?"*

Positive spirituality conversations, in fact, can follow from any of the CAMPS dimensions of spirituality that we have considered in Chapter 1. Where do people find energy and direction in the arena of spiritual community? Rituals and spiritual practices? Meaning and purpose? Passions? Connections to the Divine?

Such conversations, finally, may occur at multiple points in the process of health and wellness care... preventive visits, acute care, life transitions (like partnering and having children), chronic illness, and death and dying. We will consider specific approaches in substantial detail in Chapters 8 through 10.

Organizational soul

The third way that health and wellness care providers contribute to spiritual care is by being active members of healing organizations.

I have also suggested earlier, in the Introduction and in publications over the years,[8-10] that organizations have qualities of "soul" and that these qualities can play a significant role in the process of care and healing. Organizations that have a combination of beneficial qualities of soul, such as

- staff having a shared understanding of mission,
- staff functioning as a community or people who support one another, deal with conflicts directly, care about one another and (even) have fun, and
- leaders who provide good models of personal integrity and "bring out the best in people"

... show substantially better measures of staff satisfaction, patient satisfaction, process measures and health care outcomes than those organizations that do not.

Theologian John Shea speaks of "welcoming spiritualities," the qualities of health care organizations that extend hospitality and welcome to suffering people who come through the door.[11] If we can make our organizations places of hospitality and serenity, he suggests, we can significantly support the process of healing.

The organization where I practice... a family medicine clinic... has some staff who do an exemplary job welcoming people. The "first contact" person that patients encounter when they come in the door is a man who has been in that position for several years and who takes pride in knowing and greeting most of our patients by name… no small feat in a practice of several thousand patients. The medical assistant who works most closely with me knows the patients that I see and often greets them with enthusiasm and warmth… "Jane," she says, hugging Jane, "It's so good to see you." I sometimes suspect that this touching greeting may contribute more to people's well-being than do the incisive conversations they subsequently have with Dr. Craigie.

If organizational soul matters… if qualities of culture in organizations contribute to healing and wholeness, then anything that we can do to support the healing qualities of our organizations is a legitimate part of spiritual care. As clinicians, our roles in this process typically involve personal wholeness and integrity, leadership, and mentoring. We will explore all of this further in Chapters 11 through 13.

SUMMARY

- Spiritual care professionals can often minister significantly to the multi-layered emotions and spiritual doubts of suffering people.
- Those of us who are health and wellness care clinicians provide spiritual care…
  - by means of our intention and presence,
  - by exploring and energizing patients' spiritual values and resources, and
  - by nurturing the spiritually healing qualities of health care organizations.

REFERENCES

1. Hamdy R. Chaplains, the hidden assets. *Southern Med J.* 2006;99(6):638.
2. Daaleman T, Usher B, Williams S, Rawlings J, Hanson L. An exploratory study of spiritual care at the end of life. *Ann Fam Med.* 2008;6(5):406-411.
3. Lunn J. Spiritual care in a multi-religious context. *J Pain Palliat Care Pharmacother.* 2003;17(3-4):153-166.

4. Puchalski CM, McSkimming S. Creating healing environments: An initiative seeks to restore "heart and humanity" to depersonalized health care. *Health Progress.* 2006;87(3).

5. Puchalski CM, Lunsford B, Harris M, Miller T. Interdisciplinary spiritual care for seriously ill and dying patients: A collaborative model. *The Cancer Journal.* 2006;12(5):398-416.

6. Anandarajah G. The 3 H and BMSEST models for spirituality in multicultural whole-person medicine. *Ann Fam Med.* 2008;6(5):448-458.

7. Craigie F, Jr. Spiritual caregiving by health care professionals. *Health Progress.* 2007;88(2):61-65.

8. Craigie FC, Jr. Weaving spirituality into organizational life: Suggestions for processes and programs. *Health Prog.* Mar-Apr 1998;79(2):25-28, 32.

9. Craigie FC, Jr. The Spirit and work: Observations about spirituality and organizational life. *Journal of Psychology and Christianity.* 1999;18:43-53.

10. Craigie FC, Jr., Hobbs RF. Exploring the organizational culture of exemplary community health center practices. *Fam Med.* 2004;36(10):733-738.

11. Shea J. *Spirituality and Health care: Reaching toward a Holistic Future.* Chicago: The Park Ridge Center; 2000.

Chapter Four

Three Arenas of Spiritual Care

*I used to believe that we must choose between
science and reason on one hand,
and spirituality on the other, in how we lead our lives.
Now I consider this a false choice.
We can recover the sense of sacredness,
not just in science, but in perhaps every area of life.*[1]

Larry Dossey, MD

G*allia est omnis divisa in partes tres.* All Gaul is divided into three parts. These words, the opening line from Julius Caesar's commentaries on the Gallic Wars, are permanently emblazoned in the brains of all students of high school Latin.

So, too, spirituality in health and wellness care. I'm not sure that there is a memorable sentence that is emblazoned in our brains, but I have proposed for many years that all spirituality in care giving is divided into three parts, or arenas.[2]

As we discussed briefly in the Introduction, the large preponderance of literature about spirituality in medicine, nursing, counseling and integrative health care has focused on the approaches that we as caregivers pursue with the people whom we serve. This is the "clinical" arena, encompassing the ways that we connect with and support *what matters to our patients.* Equally important in the overall landscape of spirituality in health and wellness care are the personal arena... connecting with *what matters to us...* and the organizational arena... connecting with *the shared energy of people working together.*

When these three arenas are functioning well and harmoniously, with a) personally centered clinicians, b) exercising good clinical skills for supporting the positive spiritualities of patients, c) in health care organizations that bring out the best in one another, we see great spiritual care. When one or more of the three arenas is lacking... and I believe that the deficiency is more often in personal demoralization or organizational disempowerment than it is in inadequate clinical skills or approaches... the overall enterprise of spiritual care is lacking, as well.

THE PERSONAL ARENA

Pediatrician Robert A. Pendergrast, Jr., comments,

An integrative approach to spirituality in clinical work starts with me. I have to be a person of integrity, grounded in compassion and the intention to be a channel of healing for my patients. I may be spiritual in touching the shoulder of a struggling teen in my office, but equally spiritual in firmly confronting a person who is abusing their own body; both are acts of integrity. When I am reminded of my own spiritual vocation as a healer, then I am ready to connect to and honor the spirit of my patient. This means listening to them, opening a space for them to tell their own story, and then sharing my thoughts with them about how their story could have a better ending than they thought when they came into the exam room.

Integrity... grounded in compassion... reminded of spiritual vocation as a healer... Dr. Pendergrast says it well. I think that it does "start with us," as we discussed in the last chapter, because "intention" and "presence" are the foundational building blocks of spiritual care.

Perhaps it is possible to engage some routine and concrete tasks when we are not personally centered and grounded. Maybe you can successfully change the fuel pump on your 2001 Ford F150 or sew the backing on a quilt when you are tired, distracted, or angry. But even with concrete tasks such as these, I would argue that our personal centeredness matters. It is completely clear to me that I do a better job building a staircase, playing the fiddle, or shooting foul shots when I am more mindful and centered than when I am not.

If this is the case with concrete tasks like home repair or sewing... that our own centeredness enhances how we do things... then I think it is even more the case in the more complicated realms of human relationships.

You will note a number of words linked to the personal arena of spiritual care in the preceding paragraphs... "intention," "presence," "groundedness," "centeredness," "compassion," "vocation." These words converge in the ideas of our own personal wellness, wholeness and groundedness as we follow our calling as healers and encouragers of other people.

Our personal groundedness is important for four reasons.

Equanimity

First, our own spiritual groundedness and well-being helps us to have more of a spirit of balance and equanimity as we move through the day. The literature we have reviewed about the relationships of spirituality with coping, mindfulness, and quality of life pertains to us as caregivers as much as it does to our patients. In a world where most of us have more day to day responsibilities than we can completely discharge, we can do what we do in a way that is relatively less peaceful, or relatively more peaceful. To the extent that we draw upon our own spiritual resources, we experience... as do the cohorts of patients in the spirituality and health literature... greater personal equanimity, enhanced coping, and (probably) better health status. In addition, I would personally add to this list the observation that when we are more centered and grounded in the work we do, life is more fun.

I have a Buddhist friend who reminds me that the Dalai Lama often says that he is thankful every day for the Chinese, because they are his greatest teachers. Goodness knows the Dalai Lama has ample reason to be bitter and vindictive because of how the Chinese have treated his faith community and his country. What a remarkable perspective to be thankful for their presence in his life, to completely reframe what, to most of us, has been an egregiously unfair saga. Spiritual groundedness leads to personal equanimity.

Patient care

Second, our own spiritual groundedness helps us to provide better care to the people whom we work with.

As I write this, I have presented a conference earlier this week for our faculty, residents and students on personal resilience… summarizing and reflecting together about some of the psychological and spiritual literature on perspectives and approaches that help us to live with balance, dignity, and even joy in spite of the outside challenges that come at us. We made an inventory of some of these challenges… multiple concurrent responsibilities, productivity demands, lack of sleep, feelings of powerlessness, demanding patients… and then spoke together about our reactions. It was intriguing (but not surprising) to me that there was unanimity in the opinion that our own centeredness and groundedness makes a significant difference personally for us, and also in the care we provide. As one faculty member asked, "How can it possibly *not* make a difference?"

When I am centered and mindful, I am able to be "with people" more effectively. I pay closer and better attention to what people are saying, in words and between the lines. I notice more of the subtleties of voice tone and facial expression. I ask crisper questions. I suspect that my recall and integration of evidence-based literature is greater, and that the words and perspectives that I string together are more focused and articulate. And finally… to be less reductionistic and more integrative... I think that the energy of my presence with people is much more peaceful and healing than when I am not centered and mindful.

Openness to intuition

Third, our spiritual groundedness helps us to be more open to the wellspring of wisdom and intuition that surrounds us.

This point is made in different ways, with different language, by different people. One of the participants in my 1999 study of spirituality in family physicians said that her spiritual well-being enabled her to be more "available as an instrument of healing" in the lives of her patients. A second commented that when he was more centered, he was more "open to God's presence."

The context is that so much of what we do as healers is more of an inductive process than a deductive process. An oncology nurse recounts,

I was working with a couple where the woman had end-stage lung cancer and passed away shortly after we put her on Hospice care. The husband was devastated. I followed up with him following his wife's death and nothing that I did or said seemed to move him out of his despair. He wouldn't say much... he was really closed off into himself... but he was clearly suffering. One day, we got together at the cancer center where his wife had died and, it being a nice day, I suggested we walk in the gardens. As we strolled down the path, we came upon a dead butterfly on the ground in front of us. I picked it up and held it up to him in my open hands, saying nothing. He was just transfixed, and I could see tears forming in his eyes. He began to speak, as he began to weep, about the pain and sadness and love that he had had such a hard time giving voice to before. We found a bench and spoke together for the better part of an hour, and looking back, this was really the turning point in his process of healing.

As I tell groups, to whom I love to describe this story, I have thoroughly reviewed the psychotherapy outcome literature and

I can assure you that there is no therapeutic algorithm that says "When you are stuck working with somebody, go outside, find a dead animal and give it to them." The approach of the nurse did not follow deductively from a rule or algorithm; it was a matter of intuition and creativity.

I believe that we are more open to intuition and creative approaches when we are more spiritually centered. I think this is the point that the physicians made about being "available as an instrument of healing" and "open to God's presence;" that there is a flow of wisdom or creative energy out there that is larger than we are and that we access best when we are more mindful and centered.

Christina Puchalski echoes this point well:

Compassionate presence sets the stage for physicians to be open to their own intuition. Intuition becomes a very important part of diagnosis and treatment. While the doctor can assimilate all the facts about symptoms and presentation of illness, it is just as important to use the powers of observation and intuition to gather more data. A cough may actually be a symptom of anxiety which can be picked up if the doctor senses what is going on with the patient beyond just the words exchanged. By being fully present with patients, doctors' intuitive skills can be strengthened.[3] (p.402)

Dr. Puchalski is addressing a physician audience, but the principle applies to all of us who provide health and wellness care.

This is important because so much of what we do in health and wellness care is really more an inductive process... a matter of intuition and creativity... than it is a deductive process, in the sense of applications of rules. Even where there are clearly-defined treatment approaches and protocols, the application of those protocols often involves "art" as much as "science." For instance, there are data that cognitive-behavior therapy is the treatment of choice for most anxiety disorders and that metformin protects against the cardiovascular complications of diabetes. Referring someone for cognitive-behavior therapy or writing a script for metformin... the deductive process... is the easy part.

The challenge is what you *say* to the real person in front of you in the course of doing this. The anxious and probably depressed person who has a stressful workplace, who has maxed out their credit cards and who has daily headaches. The 287 pound woman whose blood sugars are out of control who comes from a family/cultural setting where it is normal and completely acceptable to be "big." This is the art of health and wellness care... the inductive process... the venue of intuition and inspiration.

You can run, but you can't hide

The final reason why our own spiritual groundedness and well-being matter is because the energy that we put out as we move through our days touches our colleagues and co-workers.

Quaker writer Parker Palmer speaks of the power of individuals in organizations to bring light or cast darkness upon the people around them.[4] Most of us can recall times in a workplace when a chronically angry or cynical colleague has had the ability to dampen the spirits of everyone within hailing distance, or conversely when a calm and affiming colleague has had the ability to help the organization through hard times.

I recall a British comedy routine, set in a restaurant, in which there is a strident clatter of pots and pans coming from the kitchen. The waiter, adjustuing his tie as he approaches the patrons' table, tries to give an appearance of calm. The worried patrons know otherwise. Our inner lives... which we sometimes think are hidden... show through and touch the lives of people around us.

THE CLINICAL ARENA

I saw a 50 year old woman who had just been diagnosed with breast cancer. As I spoke with her about treatment options, I asked how she was doing. She dissolved in tears... not so much, she said, about her own health as about her grown daughter. She and the daughter had had a strained relationship for years, coming to a head after some terrible arguments when the daugher was in high school. The daughter left home when she was 18 and she and my patient had not spoken in over a year. I asked what this was like for her and how she would describe why this was painful and meaningful for her. She said that she felt guilty as a mom and loved her daughter and couldn't bear the idea of dying without somehow setting things right. We talked about some ideas she had about what she could do and I commented that it seemed to me that she did indeed love her daughter very much. You could see a glimmer of pride and hope, and when she left, she held my hands in both her hands and said how much it had meant to her that I helped her to see more clearly the importance of her relationship with her daughter at this point in her life.

One can tell a host of stories about incorporating spirituality in the health and wellness care of patients. This particular story does not have specific spiritual language, but is another good example of our definition of spiritual care from the last chapter: "helping people to connect with the things that really matter to them." This physician meets the patient where she is, moves beyond purely medical care to explore the nature of her suffering, and helps to bring into focus the patient's deep and heartfelt desire to make things right with her daughter.

This is the clinical arena of spiritual care; the compassionate, present, journeying-with people in directions… as Koop says… that are "vital and sacred" for them.

For providers of health and wellness care, the two principal spiritual care roles in the clinical arena that we considered in the last chapter were a) cultivating healing intention and compassionate presence, and b) exploring and supporting positive spirituality and resources. Our *roles* as bearers of healing intention and compassionate presence pertain to *all* of the encounters that we have with the people with whom we work. The *conversation* around positive spirituality arises in a *variety of related ways* in the different settings in which we see people.

- In **wellness and preventive care,** the positive spirituality conversation might explore what people most value for their lives, where they find passion and energy, and what they take pride in.

- In *life transitions* (such as partnering, competing school, bearing children and retiring), the conversation might explore what the forthcoming changes mean to people and how they see their enduring values taking form in the next chapters into which they are entering.

- In work with **health behavior and lifestyle change,** the positive spirituality conversation might explore the life values that underlie and give energy to people's efforts to pursue healthy choices and practices.

- In *chronic illness care,* the conversation might explore the nature of people's suffering and how they can make sense of what is happening and still find meaning in the presence of whatever limitations they have.

- And in the setting of *terminal illness,* the positive spirituality conversation might explore a review of life, a reflection on legacy, and a consideration of how remaining time could be best lived with dignity and grace.

The clinical arena, of course, also involves recognizing significant spiritual *issues,* as we have discussed, and enlisting the valuable help and collaboration of our chaplain and spiritual care specialist colleagues.

THE ORGANIZATIONAL ARENA

The health center is in an urban neighborhood with its share of economic and social challenges. I go in the door and have a palpable feeling of hospitality and tranquility. The physician I speak with says that the staff are passionately committed to working there because they take great pride in providing quality care to people who really need it. She herself "could make a lot more money working in the suburbs," but finds it fulfilling and life-giving to practice there. She has worked in other practices, she says, where "the individuals were great but the feel of the whole place wasn't there." (Field notes from qualitative study of family physician interviews[5])

I recall my visit to the health center quite clearly, ten years after the fact. The neighborhood had had the regrettably common struggles with violence and drug trafficking, and revealed a landscape of generally-untended properties and broken trucks. The building was unpretentious... Nouveau Cinder Block, 1958. Inside the door, however, there really was a discernibly different spirit. Words come to mind such as "hospitality," "welcome," "peacefulness," "tranquility," "calm," and "grace."

This discernible spirit may have had to do with a number of factors. I was greeted warmly. I had scheduled my visit, but the initial contact people didn't know me from Adam (except that I guess I would have been several millennia younger). The spirit of the health center may have had to do with seeing the ways that the staff related to patients and to one another. People were happy. It may have had to do with the simple but tidy décor... some art from local children on the walls... or with the quiet and tasteful music in the background. It may have had to do with the energy of the staff... many of whom had grown up in the surrounding neighborhood... wanting to make contributions to this community.

The comments from the physician working there were remarkable. In spite of the personal financial sacrifice, she chose to be there not just because of some theoretical sense of socially responsibility... although this was certainly part of her value system... but because it was "life-giving." She had worked in other places with "great individuals," but in this practice, she found that there was a "feel of the whole place" that made it qualitatively different from other practices with similarly skilled and devoted colleagues.

The "feel of the whole place" is a good way of describing the organizational arena of spirituality in health and wellness care. As I suggested in the Introduction, there are many other linguistic frameworks for the idea of organizational spirit or soul… "atmosphere," "culture," "tone," "environment," and so forth. The underlying premise is that organizations are, as the health center physician points out, more than the sum total of the individuals who work in them. Individual clinical, administrative, or support staff can be "great," but the overall culture or soul of organizations can be life-draining or life-giving.

I believe that the organizational arena is the third essential piece of the landscape of spirituality in health and wellness care. Organizations have souls in the same way that individuals have souls; spirit is embodied in organizations in the same way that it is in individuals.

This is both good news and a challenge or those of us who practice in health and wellness care. The *good news* is that it moves us away from the responsibility of the entire burden of embodying and incorporating spirituality in the work that we do. If I practice at a health center with the organizational qualities that I have described, then I can feel comfortable that there will be some calming and affirming benefit to patients that complements whatever I do in the office. The *challenge* is that we are all players in the nurturing of organizational soul. If I am dispirited, angry, or curt, the energy underlying these qualities spreads. If I am centered and generous, the energy underlying these qualities spreads, as well.

Let's look briefly at some literature about the importance of organizational spirit or culture, and at qualities of spirited organizations.

Organizational culture matters

There are several lines of research in health care support the proposition (that the business community has discussed for many years[6-9]), that organizational culture is not a superfluous nicety, but is central to the performance and productivity of organizations.

Cross-sectional studies of organizational culture. Cross-sectional studies in this arena have looked principally at three outcome variables.

- *Staff satisfaction.* Staff perceptions of teamwork, organizational morale and collaborative norms for decision-making have been associated with job satisfaction and organizational commitment.[10, 11] Cultures of "empowerment" in health care (access to information, support, and the opportunity to develop professionally) have been associated with work satisfaction, lower levels of burnout, staff commitment, and better physical and emotional health.[12-15] Other culture variables such as "group cohesion" and leadership have been associated with favorable rates of retention and turnover.[16-18]
- *Patient satisfaction.* Not surprisingly, staff and patient satisfaction and loyalty are closely linked.[19-21] Patient satisfaction has been associated with medical/cultural variables such as "progressive participatory decision-making culture" and "teamwork culture."[22, 23]
- *Quality outcomes.*
  o *Medical process variables* such as prescription drug errors,[24] implementation of QI initiatives,[25] and adherence to ambulatory care screening guidelines[26] have been linked to cultural variables such as cohesiveness, mission orientation, teamwork, and valuing of innovation.
  o Measures of *quality of care* such as chronic disease management,[27] diabetes care,[28] and functional health and mortality[29] have been linked to organizational qualities such as shared vision and objectives, staff involvement and safety in decision-making, commitment to excellence, support for innovation, and clinician-colleague relationships.
  o And *financial parameters* have been favorably associated with cultural variables such as involvement, empowerment, trust, openness, and teamwork.[30, 31]

Intervention research and transformational narratives. Adding to cross-sectional research, there are accounts of organizational culture *interventions* (involving shared governance, reaffirmation of vision, group cohesion, teamwork, collaboration, and shared learning) that have led to institutional benefits in terms of staff and patient satisfaction, retention, and implementation of quality initiatives.[32-35]

Two multi-center national initiatives merit mention. The Fetzer Institute has conducted a major initiative in relationship-centered care that has involved a dimension of cultural transformation, moving away from internal competition and hierarchical limitations and toward values around openness, self-disclosure, genuine dialogue and collaboration.[36] And a recent report from the George Washington Institute for Spirituality and Health has described a seven-center initiative in creating "healing environments." This program finds that cultural changes in participating hospitals… associated with stronger teamwork, sense of community, and interdisciplinary relationships among staff… result in an enhanced ability to respond to the needs of patients.[37]

Exemplary practice research. Another line of research identifies exemplary units of clinical care and explores the qualities that make them work well. With my colleague Rick Hobbs, MD, I used qualitative content analysis and field observation methodologies to explore the salient characteristics of exemplary community health centers in Maine.[38] We found consistent references from staff about a sustaining and energetic "spirit," "atmosphere" and "tone" in the community of workplace relationships.

Similarly, a group from the Dartmouth Medical School has conducted extensive analysis of twenty of the best-value, best-quality clinical microsystems in North America and identified nine characteristics associated with their successes.[39] Among these characteristics are qualities of leadership (maintaining organizational focus on mission, empowering individuals and forming positive culture) and qualities of culture ("where everyone matters").

Intuition. Finally, I suggest that "truth" comes to us not only through randomized clinical trials, but also through anthropological and ethnographic approaches[40] and even through meditation and intuition.[41] In the spirit of such approaches, one may consider; *if you are a doctor... or nurse, acupuncturist, fitness instructor, nutritionist, counselor... spending over half of your waking hours at work, what kind of culture do you want to work in, that feeds your soul and brings forth the best that you can offer?*

Characteristics of soulful organizations

This literature suggests several recurring themes about positive organizational culture:

Mission. There is a shared and vital understanding that people are working together toward a meaningful purpose. An understanding of mission resides not in glitzy statements on the wall, but in the daily life and conversation of staff. In the Maine community health centers, the staff... from physicians to records clerks... said with one voice (albeit different words) that their mission was to provide accessible, quality health care to underserved people. Shared understanding of a meaningful purpose gives direction to planning and decision-making, and energizes the ways that employees bring heart and soul to the workplace, beyond just being physically present.

Community. Staff in soulful organizations are not merely co-workers... co-located workers... they are a community. Being a community involves a number of types of interaction and relationships:

- *Collaboration and "helping out."* Staff in the exemplary health centers continually explore effective systems for working together and freely "lend a hand" beyond their individual job descriptions. A practice manager tells about answering phones when the front desk staff are overwhelmed. A physician assistant tells about everyone in the building working together... doctor included... to disinfect the exam tables at the end of the day.

- *Caring and knowing.* Staff frequently use the word "family" to describe their relationships. They collectively know and care about whose partner has a serious illness, and whose special needs child is graduating from high school.
- *Trust.* Staff have above-boards and respectful conversations about challenging issues.
- *Fun.* Being a community means not just resolute movement toward noble goals, but also times of celebration, laughter and joy.

Leadership. There is no dearth of resource material on leadership. One can peruse the shelves of the local bookseller and find treatises on leadership from sports coaches, politicians, religious gurus, business tycoons, generals (living and dead) and assorted pundits. In the literature of organizational culture, leadership embraces such qualities as:

- Leading by example[42] and tending to one's own spiritual well-being.[43]
- Inspiring shared vision.[43]
- Creating a culture where "everyone matters"[44] and everyone is "brought into the conversation."[42] In the health centers, weekly staff meetings (professional and support staff together) provide a remarkably egalitarian and apparently safe opportunity for people to raise issues or speak anything on their minds.
- Creating an environment where the focus is not on "management" and "direction," but on the ability of work groups to learn, adapt and self-organize.[45]

THREE INTERLOCKING PIECES

As I suggested in the Introduction, I believe that all three arenas are vital parts of the larger picture of spirituality in health and wellness care. Spiritual care is incomplete without attention to personal spirituality, as well as clinical approaches, as well as organizational soul. Take one in isolation... a common example being good clinical skills in dis-spirited practitioners or disempowering organizations... and the challenges of providing good spiritual care over time become formidable and prohibitive.

Stated positively, spiritual care can be profoundly meaningful in the setting of positive intention and centeredness among practitioners, with good clinical skills, in organizations that affirm and bring out the best in patients and staff.

Not only are these three arenas of spiritual care important, moreover, but they influence each other:

Each of the three arenas of spiritual care influences, and is influenced by, the other two, representing six possible combinations (or perhaps they are they permutations... I need to find my high school math notes.)

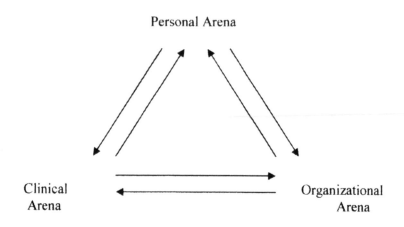

Personal Arena

Clinical
Arena

Organizational
Arena

- Personal > Clinical. Personal centeredness makes for good clinical care.
- Clinical > Personal. Sacred moments in relating to patients contribute to our personal centeredness.
- Personal > Organizational. Individual qualities and behavior influence health care teams.
- Organizational > Personal. Organizational policies and culture influence individuals.
- Organizational > Clinical. Supportive, mission-driven health care teams provide good clinical care.
- Clinical > Organizational. Episodes of collaborative and spiritually sensitive care strengthen teamwork.

A couple of examples. An oncology nurse recounts how clinical events can touch us personally and touch the teams with whom we work:

I was working late one day, probably making out coverage schedules, when an elderly man whom we had worked with for several months came up to the nursing station. I knew from the recent reports that he was not doing well and he really looked like he was having a lot of trouble getting around. I went around the counter and put my arm on his shoulder... told him I was so glad to see him. I asked him how I could help him... I was puzzled because this was long after the medical staff had left for the day. He looked me in the eye and said that he knew he didn't have long to live and he just had wanted to come by to let us all know how much it had meant to him that we had "treated him like a man." I'm not sure I said anything terribly important back to him, but I remember giving him a hug and feeling the warmth and energy of his thin, bony embrace. I told my staff the next day and there were more than a few tears as we talked for a few minutes about taking care of him.

A fitness instructor describes how individuals and health care teams influence one another, as well.

All of us had been pretty bummed out for months. The director was always on our case. We never had enough people in our classes, we weren't developing new programs, we weren't recruiting new members, we were sitting around too much. A couple of staff who worked fewer hours than the rest of us were let go without much of any warning or explanation, which made the rest of us edgy. Then, miracle of miracles, he left. I don't know where he went and I don't particularly care. The Board replaced him with a woman whose main connection with the organization was that she had been an active and faithful customer. I was so impressed at what a difference she made. She spent the first few weeks just having long conversations and getting to know each of the three or four dozen employees. With me, she was really interested in why I was doing this work and what gave me joy and what I thought I best could contribute. We started to have staff meetings where everybody really had a chance to say what was on their minds… it was two-way, which we had never had before. She has a great sense of humor and she spends a lot of the day out in the public areas mixing it up with customers and staff. She's not dictatorial at all, but she makes us want to do good work… she reminds us why we're in this business, to promote the health and well-being of people in our community.

The "interlocking" relationships among these three arenas of spirituality are important because they give us multiple pathways by which we can make a difference in providing spiritual care. You can tend to your own spiritual well-being, cultivate some good clinical skills, and contribute positively to the health care team of which you are a part… and anticipate with some confidence that your life and those of your patients and colleagues will be enriched as a result.

The remainder of this book will explore how this happens.

SUMMARY

- The larger picture of spirituality in health and wellness care is comprised of three vital and interrelated arenas; a personal arena, a clinical arena, and an organizational arena.

- When all three arenas are functioning well and harmoniously, with a) personally centered clinicians, b) exercising good clinical spiritual care skills, c) in health care organizations that bring out the best in one another, we see great spiritual care.
- The *personal* arena of spiritual care has to do with the centeredness and groundedness of clinicians. The personal spiritual well-being of clinicians is important because:
  o It promotes a personal spirit of equanimity.
  o It enhances patient care.
  o It helps clinicians to be open to intuition.
  o The energy we put out as we move through our days touches our colleagues and co-workers.
- The *clinical* arena of spiritual care involves cultivating healing intention and compassionate presence, and exploring and supporting what is "vital and sacred" in patients' lives. Substantial work with spiritual *issues* often falls in the domain of our spiritual care colleagues.
- Our conversations about patients' spiritual values and resources arise in a variety of settings, including
  o Wellness and preventive care
  o Life transitions
  o Health behavior and lifestyle change
  o Chronic illness care
  o Terminal illness
- The *organizational* arena of spiritual care has to do with qualities of organizational culture and leadership… soul… that affirm and bring out the best in employees, and support compassionate and skilled care for patients.
- Substantial research points to the conclusion that organizational culture matters. Support for this proposition comes from
  o Cross-sectional studies of organizational culture
  o Intervention research and transformational narratives
  o Exemplary practice research
  o Intuition

- Characteristics of soulful organizations include
  - Mission
  - Community
  - Empowering leadership
- What happens in each of the three arenas of spiritual care... personal, clinical and organizational... influences what happens in the other two.

REFERENCES

1. Dossey L. *Reinventing Medicine: Beyond Mind-Body to a New Era of Healing.* New York: HarperOne; 2000.
2. Craigie FC, Jr. The Spirit and work: Observations about spirituality and organizational life. *Journal of Psychology and Christianity.* 1999;18:43-53.
3. Puchalski CM, Lunsford B, Harris M, Miller T. Interdisciplinary spiritual care for seriously ill and dying patients: A collaborative model. *The Cancer Journal.* 2006;12(5):398-416.
4. Palmer P. Leading from within. In: Conger J, ed. *Spirit at Work: Discovering the Spirituality in Leadership.* San Francisco: Jossey-Bass; 1994.
5. Craigie FC, Jr., Hobbs RF, 3rd. Spiritual perspectives and practices of family physicians with an expressed interest in spirituality. *Fam Med.* Sep 1999;31(8):578-585.
6. Chappell T. *The Soul of a Business.* New York: Bantam; 1993.
7. Owen H. *The Power of Spirit: How Organizations Transform.* San Francisco: Berrett-Koehler; 2000.
8. Briskin A. *The Stirring of Soul in the Workplace.* San Francisco: Berrett-Koehler; 1998.
9. Toms M, ed. *The Soul of Business.* Carlsbad, CA: New Dimensions Foundation; 1997.
10. Sikorska-Simmons E. Organizational culture and work-related attitudes among staff in assisted living. *J Gerontol Nurs.* 2006;32(2):19-27.
11. Campbell S, Fowles E, Weber B. Organizational structure and job satisfaction in public health nursing. *Public Health Nurs.* 2004;21(6):564-571.
12. Laschinger H, Finegan J, Shamian J. The impact of workplace

empowerment, organizational trust on staff nurses' work satisfaction and organizational commitment. *Health Care Manage Rev.* 2001;26(3):7-23.

13. Laschinger H, Almost J, Tuer-Hodes D. Workplace empowerment and magnet hospital characteristics: Making the link. *J Nurs Admin.* 2003;33(7-8):410-422.

14. Laschinger H, Almost J, Purdy N, Kim J. Predictors of nurse managers' health in Canadian restructured healthcare settings. *Can J Nurs Leadership.* 2004;17(4):88-105.

15. Sarmiento T, Laschinger H, Iwasiw C. Nurse educators' workplace empowerment, burnout, and job satisfaction: Testing Kantor's theory. *J Adv Nurs.* 2004;46(2):134-143.

16. Anthony M, Standing T, Glick J, Duffy M, et al. Leadership and nurse retention: The pivotal role of nurse managers. *J Nurs Adm.* 2005;35(3):146-155.

17. Karsh B, Booske B, Sainfort F. Job and organizational determinants of nursing home employee commitment, job satisfaction and intent to turnover. *Ergonomics.* 2005;48(10):1260-1281.

18. Shader K, Broome M, Broome C, West M, Nash M. Factors influencing satisfaction and anticipated turnover for nurses in an academic medical center. *J Nurs Adm.* 2001;31(4):210-216.

19. Atkins P, Marshall B, Javalgi R. Happy employees lead to loyal patients. Survey of nurses and patients shows a strong link between employee satisfaction and patient loyalty. *J Health Care Mark.* 1996;16(4):14-23.

20. Vahey D, Aiken L, Sloane D, Clarke S, Vargas D. Nurse burnout and patient satisfaction. *Med Care.* 2004;42(2 Suppl):II57-66.

21. Geyer S. Hand in hand: Patient and employee satisfaction. *Trustee.* 2005;58(6):12-14,19,11.

22. Meterko M, Mohr D, Young G. Teamwork culture and patient satisfaction in hospitals. *Med Care.* 2004;42(5):492-498.

23. Rondeau K, Wagar T. Nurse and resident satisfaction in magnet long-term care organizations: Do high involvement approaches matter? *J Nurs Manag.* 2006;14(3):244-250.

24. Shortell S, Jones R, Rademaker A, Gillies R, et al. Assessing the impact of total quality management and organizational culture on multiple outcomes of care for coronary artery bypass graft surgery patients. *Med Care.* 2000;38(2):207-217.

25. Parker V, Wubbenhorst W, Young G, Desai K, et al. Implementing quality improvement in hospitals: The role of leadership and culture. *Am J Med Qual.* 1999;14(1):64-69.

26. Vaughn T, McCoy K, BootsMiller B, Woolson R, et al. Organizational predictors of adherence to ambulatory care screening guidelines. *Med Care.* 2002;40(12):1172-1185.

27. Bower P, Campbell S, Bojke C, Sibbald B. Team structure, team climate and the quality of care in primary care: An observational study. *Qual Saf Health Care.* 2003;12:273-279.

28. Campbell SM, Hann M, Hacker J, et al. Identifying predictors of high quality care in English general practice: An observational study. *BMJ.* 2001;323:784ff.

29. Safran D, Miller W, Beckman H. Organizational dimensions of relationship-centered care: Theory, evidence and practice. *J Gen Intern Med.* 2006;21(Suppl 1):S9-15.

30. Harmon J, Scotti D, Behson S, Farias G, et al. Effects of high-involvement work systems on employee satisfaction and service costs in veterans healthcare. *J Healthcare Manag.* 2003;48(6):393-406.

31. Shortell S, Schmittdiel J, Wang M, Li R, et al. An empirical assessment of high-performing medical groups: Results from a national study. *Med Care Res Tev.* 2005;62(4):407-434.

32. Baker C, Beglinger J, King S, Salyards M, et al. Transforming negative work cultures: A practical strategy. *J Nurs Adm.* 2000;30(7/8):357-363.

33. Malloch K. A total healing environment: the Yavapai Regional Medical Center story. *J Healthcare Manag.* Nov-Dec 1999;44(6):495-512.

34. Odwazny R, Hasler S, Abrams R, McNutt R. Organizational and cultural changes for providing safe patient care. *Qual Manag Health Care.* 2005;14(3):132-143.

35. Force M. Creating a culture of service excellence: Empowering nurses within the shared governance councilor model. *Health Care Manag (Frederick).* 2004;23(3):262-266.

36. Malloch K, Sluyter D, Moore N. Relationship-centered care: Achieving true value in healthcare. *J Nurs Adm.* 2000;30(7/8):379-385.

37. Puchalski C, McSkimming S. Creating healing environments. *Health Prog.* 2006;87(3):30-35.

38. Craigie FC, Jr., Hobbs RF. Exploring the organizational culture of exemplary community health center practices. *Fam Med.* 2004;36(10):733-738.

39. Nelson EC, Batalden PB, Huber TP, et al. Microsystems in health care: Part 1. Learning from high-performing front-line clinical units. *Jt Comm J Qual Improv.* Sep 2002;28(9):472-493.

40. Barry C. The role of evidence in alternative medicine: Contrasting biomedical and anthropological approaches. *Soc Sci Med.* 2006;62:2646-2657.

41. Levin J. The power of love. *Alt Ther.* 1999;5(4):79-86.

42. Whyte D. Making work meaningful. In: Harris G, ed. *Body & soul.* New York: Kensington; 1999.

43. Strack G, Fottler MD. Spirituality and effective leadership in healthcare: Is there a connection? *Front Health Serv Manage.* Summer 2002;18(4):3-18.

44. Huber TP, Godfrey MM, Nelson EC, Mohr JJ, Campbell C, Batalden PB. Microsystems in health care: Part 8: Developing people and improving work life: What front-line staff told us. *Joint Commission Journal on Quality and Safety.* 2003;29(10):512-522.

45. McDaniel R, Driebe D. Complexity science and health care management. *Adv Health Care Mgmt.* 2001;2:11-36.

NINE PRACTICAL APPROACHES TO BRINGING POSITIVE SPIRITUALITY INTO HEALTH AND WELLNESS CARE

I hope that the material that you have read or perused so far (to be quite frank, I do more perusing than reading of books myself) has stimulated for you some practical thoughts about spirituality in health and wellness care. Now, however, we will specifically turn our attention to practical approaches. If the conversation in the preceding chapters has been anchored in the questions, "What" (are we talking about) and "Why" (is this important), the conversation in the remaining chapters will be anchored in the question, "How" (can clinicians make spirituality a practical and positive part of care).

The nine practical approaches, as you will see, are divided among the personal, clinical and organizational arenas of spiritual care. For each of these arenas, we will consider three core approaches, with a large collection of practical suggestions, examples and specific strategies. The following chapters are not sequential; you can explore them as the spirit moves... which I assume you were going to do anyway. I would suggest that you experiment with the suggested strategies, or make up your own. In the same way that patients change more as a result of doing than thinking, I think that most of us develop our skills and enhance our repertoires by trying things out. See what fits for you. I want you to feel affirmed in your own style of what you do already, and I invite you to explore some new approaches, as well.

PERSONAL: CONNECTIONS WITH WHAT MATTERS TO YOU

The following three chapters explore the personal arena. The overarching idea, as we have discussed, is that our own centeredness, intention and presence represent good spiritual care and provide the foundation for more specific spiritual approaches. We will consider the roles and approaches of personal purpose and mission (Chapter 5), qualities of character (Chapter 6), and cultivating healing intention and presence (Chapter 7).

Chapter Five

Stay Connected with Your Purpose

Don't ask what the world needs; ask what makes you come alive and go do it. Because what the world needs is people who have come alive.

Howard Thurman, American theologian and civil rights activist

Why do you do what you do in health and wellness care? How did you come to be a nurse, a naturopath, a physician, a drug and alcohol counselor, a nutritionist, a life coach, or whatever it is that describes your professional role? Why has it mattered to you to do *this work*, rather than some other work? Where is the energy, the life, and the satisfaction in the work that you do?

SPIRITUAL ALIVENESS

I have always loved Thurman's idea of *coming alive*. It is akin to the observation in Chapter One from John the Apostle that spirit "gives life." The passage from death to aliveness is a fundamentally spiritual journey; doing work that makes us come alive is a spiritual path.

I presented some seminars a number of years ago about spirituality for leaders from the business community. The sessions explored what spirituality meant to them in their various entrepreneurial ventures. I recall one participant, a woman who was the CEO of an investment firm, commenting that she was realizing that "I just can't afford to have workers who are spiritually dead." Not just that it was *unpleasant* to have workers who were spiritually dead, mind you, but that she could not *afford* this in her business. She went on to say that she was realizing that qualities of enthusiasm and passion about work were profoundly important to the success of her organization.

We have all known workers… patients, colleagues, friends… who have been spiritually dead. Perhaps this quality has touched our own lives at some point. I saw a patient a few months ago who made a good living from a financial point of view working for a telecommunications firm. She was, however, completely disconnected from any sense of meaningful work. "I'm just pushing paper around my desk," she said, "not doing anything good for anybody, just putting money in the pockets of people I can't stand." She has since made some career changes that bring her more sense of satisfaction from providing support and direction to people at transition points in their lives.

Aliveness is very different.

Britney is one of the most devoted people I've ever met. She doesn't make a whole lot of money as a CNA, and her job, working here with Alzheimer's patients, isn't particularly glamorous, but you can see that she really loves what she does… she's passionate about her work. She'll tell you that anything she can do to make her patients feel more comfortable or less fearful… more loved, really… brings her incredible joy. She's not Mother Teresa… she's not perfect and she gets stressed like the rest of us… but there's this core of real devotion and passion about caring for these people.

Aliveness is conceptually related to the other qualities that we have considered that frame spiritual well-being… groundedness, centeredness, wholeness, and so forth… all of which are important to us as clinicians. As we discussed in the last chapter, these qualities of our own personal well-being

- promote a spirit of equanimity and resilience,
- help us to provide quality clinical care,
- enable us to be open to intuition, and
- spread in a ripple effect to other people with whom we work.

What the world needs… what health and wellness care needs… is people who have come alive.

ALIVENESS AND PURPOSE

Spiritual aliveness for us as caregivers is typically anchored in purpose. When we have a present awareness of doing what we do because it is meaningful… because it relates to a purpose that matters to us… we are more alive.

In my research with exemplary community health centers,[1] the methodology included interviewing all of the staff, both professional staff and support staff, and exploring why their organizations were such great places to work and to be a patient. One of the questions in our interview protocol was "Why is it important for you to work here?" In both health center sites (both in rural Maine communities), the overwhelming majority of the staff said "We are providing quality health care to people who would not otherwise have access to health care." I heard this from the physicians, the administrators, the nurses, the receptionists, the medical records clerks, the housekeepers… everyone was truly on the same page that this was what they were about as an organization and as staff working together. It was clear that this shared purpose really helped to energize and coalesce them as health care teams.

The practical challenge is to maintain the present awareness of purpose. There are countless influences in health and wellness care that compete for our time, attention, and energy, such as productivity requirements, managed care authorization, endless paperwork, and multiple concurrent responsibilities. It is easy for purpose to become lost in the shuffle. However, if aliveness is important because it supports the personal arena of spiritual care (by means of equanimity, clinical care, and so forth), and if purpose is a foundation for aliveness, then the commitment to cultivate a present sense of purpose is a vital and practical part of good spiritual care. The first practical approach: Stay connected with your purpose.

STAYING CONNECTED WITH PURPOSE

I want to suggest two particular approaches that support the present awareness of purpose.

The origin story

In a world where the daily demands tend to obscure the larger picture of what we are doing, revisiting the origins of our commitment to our work can provide a re-orienting and re-invigoration to purpose. How did you come to do what you are doing? Why are you a provider of health and wellness care instead of a manager of a hedge fund? Why did you pass up the comfortable opportunity to be the vice president in the family business in order to go to school for seven years to be a naturopath? Aren't there easier way to make a living than putting up with the increasing work demands and nights and weekends of being a nurse? What was it that originally gave you the energy and passion to be a family therapist?

Stories have power, and the historical review of our own journeys doing what we do is best visited in story form.

Two examples. First, I want to share with you some of my own journey in becoming a psychologist with the interests and passions that I have. Second, I will show you a great archival example of an origin story from a physician colleague.

Fred's origin story

I am a child of the sixties. As a lifelong addict of major league baseball, one of my earlier fond memories is following the Maris/Mantle quest to break Babe Ruth's single-season home run record in the summer of 1961. Maris was successful on the last day of the season, as his solo home run off of Tracy Stallard beat the Red Sox one to nothing and introduced the infamous asterisk to the record book. Yes, it was the 61st home run, but no, it was not within Ruth's 154 games, so it was forever tainted.

As the decade wore on, the Vietnam War captured the nation's attention and, increasingly, its grief. I followed the tumultuous events of 1968… the assassinations, the Johnson withdrawal, the emergence of Eugene McCarthy, the Democratic convention, the election of Richard Nixon… with careful attention and, mostly, a heavy heart.

My own personal response was to throw myself into community work, spending most of the summer of 1968 working at the Solid Rock Baptist Church in Paterson, New Jersey. The Solid Rock Baptist Church was in an urban neighborhood that was fifteen miles away and a world apart from my tidy suburban home. Dozens of paper fans bearing the image of Martin Luther King honored the memory of Dr. King but did little to attenuate the discomfort of the mid-Atlantic heat and humidity. My role was to help out with a daytime activity program for younger school-age children; I remember trucking in supplies for creative art projects and staging kickball games amid the debris of inner-city life. The shopping cart was First Base, the truck tire was Second Base, the pile of sheetrock was Third Base. Home was probably somebody's hat.

I went to Dartmouth College with the assumption that I would major in Government. I think I joined in the political consciousness of the times and thought that perhaps I could work in the arena of community organization and governance to make the world a better place.

Then I took a Psychology course. I was captivated. How do we know what we know? Why is it that what we perceive is always more than the sum total and objective architecture of the sensations that come to us? How do you get pigeons to dance counter-clockwise on one foot? Why do people behave in altruistic ways? Under what conditions will they lie? How is it that a neighborhood of people can hear a woman screaming and not react?

I had been a dutiful scientist in high school... I could calculate the path of a projectile and explain abiogenesis and I think I probably once knew what Avogadro's Number was and why it is important... but here was science in a dynamic relationship with social science. An empirical inquiry about people. Exploration of the principles under girding human life, directed toward the same hope I had had for several years of ultimately working to make the world a better place.

I immersed myself in the field. Courses, tutorials, late afternoon conversations with professors, research. I did an honors project evaluating the proposition that it would be reinforcing for fourth-grade children to be imitated. If this project still exists, I suspect I can say with assurance that no one has thought about it, much less looked at it, in the intervening 37 years.

The spring of 1970 presented particular challenges for the country and for college communities. Fueled by the Cambodia invasion and the Kent State deaths, student strikes spread widely. The strike movement at Dartmouth had the character of a Garrison Keillor novel... earnest people who didn't quite connect all of the dots. The leaders of the movement had visions of following the path of their Columbia University comrades in bringing academic life to a standstill to urge forward the shared revolution of the people, from the oppressed masses overseas to the cafeteria ladies and janitors in our midst. They overtook the President's office and vowed to remain there until the revolution had been accomplished. Unfortunately for the movement, the cafeteria ladies and janitors were not much interested, not wanting to compromise their employment, and the President invited the protestors to stay as long as they wished, make themselves some coffee and please turn off the lights whenever they were done.

For me, the most powerful memories of that time came from off-campus canvassing. Several dozen people who were willing to go to homes in the community on behalf of an antiwar petition gathered in the Psychology building for an orientation to canvassing presented by one of the senior faculty. Dress like people in the community, show respect, listen to what they have to say. Armed with these pieces of advice and sheaves of petitions, we headed out.

Looking back across the years, I have no specific recollection of my canvassing conversations with people with one exception. Driving through rural dairy country, I approached a farmstead where there was a man outside the barn, looking to be finishing up end-of-the-day chores. I pulled in, parking next to the Farmall, waved and came up to speak with him. Middle-aged, skin wrinkled from life outdoors, Carter's bib overalls. With my jeans, I didn't dress exactly like him, but it was close enough.

I introduced myself and explained why I was there, describing my concern about the war and the suffering that it had brought upon American and Vietnamese people. He responded that he had been in the infantry in the Korean War, fighting in grinding, cold, gruesome battles. Friends of his had died in vicious combat at Chosin Reservoir. These experiences had left him, he said, with the belief that Asian people were something less than human, and he found it hard to be at all sympathetic to their suffering… so, no, he would not be signing my petition.

This opinion was, of course, blatantly racist. It seemed to me, though, that it really was not my place to say this and, in fact, I realized that I was much less interested in changing his mind than I was in understanding the pain in his life that had led him to such a place of bitterness and sadness. We spoke for a few minutes… hearing more of his story… and I suppose at some point I said a few words about my motivation and my hopes. We shook hands and he wished me well. As I pulled back out on to the road, I thought of the professor's advice about respect and listening. I didn't agree with his conclusions, but it was humbling to consider what it would be like to have been him.

I applied to graduate school and had the good fortune to be accepted, in an environment where the interest in positions considerably exceeded the availability of positions. With my faithful parents providing support and driving back-up, I took my 3-speed, non-air-conditioned Plymouth Duster across the country to Salt Lake City, Utah, to begin my studies.

Growing out of my community and college experience with children, I pictured myself pursuing a career in patenting education and child management. My advisor had been a student of Gerald Patterson, at that time the most distinguished researcher and teacher about parenting and child management approaches in the country. With a cadre of fellow devotees, we learned the core principles of the field; ignoring misbehavior, catching children in the act of being good, and gradually teaching and shaping behavioral repertoires. I taught a parenting class at a local community center, years before I had children myself, and was astonished (as I remain astonished) that people actually attended over the course of several sessions.

My initial clinical experience in my entire career was in a behavior management practicum. Pairs of students in the class lugged extraordinarily cumbersome early-generation video equipment to the homes of families that had signed up at a community mental health center for parenting education. The idea was to videotape a "before" and "after" clip of how parents interacted with their children around structured tasks. Making a number of wrong turns on poorly-marked rural roads, my colleague and I eventually came to the trailer and rabbit farm where 6-year-old Benny and his family lived. We set up the equipment and asked the parents to have Benny do a writing task. Benny's attention, unfortunately, was somewhere else. With the parents becoming increasingly frustrated, the session quickly degenerated, with the father roughly pushing poor Benny into his chair and screaming at him... WRITE YOUR NAME! A "B," AND AN "E," AND AN "N-N-Y!"

Reviewing the tape later when he was visiting Salt Lake, Dr. Patterson called this the most extreme example of suppressive attention he had ever seen. Ah, a good start to Dr. Craigie's clinical career. Needless to say, this was the only session with Benny's family, and I can only hope that Benny is out there somewhere and making out OK.

In the summer of 1975, I began two years of internships in the Veterans Administration system. I was interested in broadening my clinical skills and, frankly, the prospect of a tax-free stipend of $8000 a year was almost too good to believe. The first year was at the VA facility in Togus, Maine, which turned out to provide my introduction to the state that has now been my home for all but two years of the intervening time. Togus, by the way, lays claim to being the oldest VA in the United States, by virtue of it being the first Old Soldier's home established shortly after the end of the Civil War. To this day, a lovely rural site and a collection of professionals that provide good clinical care. The second year was back in Salt Lake City, at a pilot substance abuse program that treated alcoholics (mostly a World War II and Korea cohort) and addicts (mostly a Vietnam cohort) together.

I quickly came to an important realization. There are no veterans who are children. Having occupied most of my clinical training up to that point with small people who had emotional struggles and made up a lot of stories, it was a new horizon to work with large people who had emotional struggles and had real stories to tell.

Frank was around 30 at the time, having grown up on the wrong side of the tracks on the fringes of Salt Lake City and often having been in modest trouble. His family had not expressed much interest in him and he had often heard that he was fundamentally no good and would never amount to anything. He escaped this emotionally-vacant upbringing by being a reasonably good tight end on the high school football team and then by enlisting in the Army as soon as he was eligible. Amid the terrors of Vietnam, the other men in his platoon provided a fellowship he had not experienced before. He learned to be tough. He learned not to feel. He learned not to be vulnerable. His high school alcohol habit was substantially supplemented by the use of marijuana and an assortment of harder drugs.

In the years since his discharge, he had held and lost a dozen jobs, settling in modestly well as a foreman of a drilling and blasting company before he was arrested for felony possession of cocaine. The plea bargain was that he would complete our substance abuse treatment program and a substantial probation as an alternative to serving time in jail.

Our initial meeting revealed a stark picture of the challenges that lay ahead. He would need to deal with the physical challenge of abstinence, finding ways to deal with the cravings that he knew would come at his most fragile times. He would need to change his friends if *he was ever to escape the culture of drug use. He would need to find new ways to occupy and structure the hours of his days. More than this, he realized that his life-long pattern of keeping other people and his own emotions at a distance was not working. He would need to find ways to let other people in, and to experience his emotions rather than covering them up with drugs.*

His hope and motivation lay in a wife who had tenaciously stood by him, and in an 18 month old son… for whom he wanted to be the father that he, himself, had never had.

Over the next month, Frank made remarkable effort and strides. He began to relate to the other men in the program with conversation that did not center around "drug talk." He gave and received honest feedback in therapy groups. As he progressed in the program, he assumed leadership among his veteran comrades, helping men new in the program to develop their own goals and supporting them along the way. He used passes to experiment with drug-free activities. He reaffirmed with his wife their commitment to make it work, together.

He graduated from the program and, when I moved on to other things several months later, was still doing well in aftercare.

My work with Frank was a pivotal experience for me. I'm not sure I gave him particularly meaningful advice… what, after all, could I really say as a non-drug-dependent mid-twenties graduate student… but I realized that my role with Frank was not as much to be a wise answer-man as it was to be an honest and caring companion on his journey. I felt privileged and honored to be let in to the intimacies of his healing journey. The grief about years lost. The pain of change. The beauty of his holding hands with his wife as they pictured their future together and with their son.

I remember Frank from time to time when my thoughts turn to why I am doing what I am doing. I think that my time with him set the tone and direction of my professional work with people since then. Journeying with people. Being present with respect and with honesty. Seeing and encouraging the best that is in people. Trying to make the world a better place in the healing and growth into fullness of life of one person at a time.

A family doctor's origin story

I wish I had kept a diary as a child. I have wonderful but vague memories of childhood, sprinkled with more vivid highlights such as playing the turkey with the Big Black Hat in 2nd grade. Had I kept a diary, I could read about when I first decided to be a doctor. I had decided medicine would be a fine career when I was a college freshman, even though I didn't know any doctors other than the man who froze the planar wart on my thumb. By the time I graduated from college and after completing all the pre-med coursework, I had no intention of going to medical school. What I do remember, without diary assistance, is what brought me back to medicine, and this time with meaning.

In Africa as a Peace Corps volunteer, I appreciated how a doctor with an interest in improving community health could make an impact on people's lives. I was involved in community projects addressing the HIV/AIDS epidemic, focusing on condom distribution, teen education, and home-based care training for families and villagers. Physicians were a rarity, and I didn't encounter any docs while working in Africa. But after two years, it was clear to me that with more medical training and a better understanding of health and disease, I could be much more creative with the limited resources available and a greater asset to the communities with which I was involved.

When I returned to the US and to my native state of Maine, I was hired at a sexual assault support center. I worked closely with police officers, district attorneys, survivors of sexual assault, and health care professionals on an interdisciplinary project aimed at improving the community response to sexual violence. In this role, I had more contact with doctors, in the ED with someone who had been assaulted or in meetings working on hospital protocols. There were appreciable differences with the project when physicians were involved. Our protocols passed readily through the approval process, we attracted more buy-in from other professionals, and we had greater ease organizing education sessions for health care professionals on managing the fallout from sexual violence. At the time, I wasn't comfortable with the power and status that physicians appeared to wield in the community, but when I witnessed the community motivation that could be sparked by doctors, I was inspired.

So I applied and was fortunately accepted to medical school. What a great tool to have in my backpack, I thought. How much more I could do to improve community health as a physician. During the first two years, I struggled with the lack of time allotted to the type of activities that brought me to medical school. I kept a focus on the community, by being a resource for students struggling with emotional or other issues and by volunteering at a local free clinic, but I wanted to focus more on the sorts of endeavors that I thought would transform me into the doctor I hoped to become. It wasn't until my 3rd year of school that I began thinking about which field of medicine would offer me the training and environment to develop into the doctor I had envisioned before applying to medical school. I enjoyed every clinical rotation of my 3rd year, but when I spent two months doing family medicine, the pieces began to fall into place. I realized then that the majority of physicians whom I considered mentors were family doctors. Beyond the scope of their medicine, which both intimidates and invigorates me, there is a focus on the community, a respect for the idea that health is more than the individual. The commitment I've seen in family medicine to patients, families, and communities reflects the values that brought me to consider medicine as a career.

What I am looking for in a residency program is a chance to learn the practice of medicine in an environment that values academic and clinical growth, commits itself to the community in which it is based, offers diverse clinical and public health opportunities, and invests itself into the well-being of its residents. From what I have experienced, Maine-Dartmouth Family Practice Residency is all of these things. It is a place where I feel confident that I will develop into an excellent clinician, a dedicated advocate for those in need, and an agent for important community and social change.

There you have it. Two different takes on the origin story. The first is quite long… thanks for being a good sport if you read through it… but I wrote it specifically for this purpose. I will suggest that you do this as an exercise and I thought it would be a good exercise for me, presenting this idea to you, to do it myself.

I believe that you learn by writing. When you put words to paper (in the laptop age, an archaic concept, but you know what I mean), the words have an ability to take life and move you in directions you may not have anticipated. I recall a conversation with an accomplished poet about her writing. Publication and communicating with other people were secondary, she said; the main reason for writing poetry was "to learn something about yourself."

In fact, I have had a couple of observations from writing this origin story. First, I deliberately tried to anchor the running narrative in particular events; specific, colorful events. I thought… and this turned out to be the case… that this rich-to-the-senses recounting of the story would help to bring forth emotions which, like words as I have suggested above, also have an ability to take life and move you in directions you may not have anticipated.

Second, I realized as I was writing the Frank vignette, which I had not intended, that this brought forth the themes about "why I am doing what I am doing." Somehow Frank appeared as I allowed the story to unfold, and I realized that my relationship with him really did form and embody some of the core values that have remained with me.

The physician story is different. I have said this is "archival;" it is a personal statement from this person's application for residency training. Senior medical students write these statements as part of the packet of material they send when they seek residency positions with our program. As I work with residents over the course of their training, I sometimes will dig out the personal statements and show them to the residents when they are getting close to graduation. Interesting reactions. Commonly, there is some eye-rolling and chuckling as the now-veterans of three years of grueling post-graduate medical education look back at what they said as fresh-faced rookies. But, equally commonly, this changes; I see some real familiarity and connection with the values about medicine that they realize are still there. I think that the spirituality of these stories has an energy that pulls people back in. With this physician, for instance, the idea that "health is more than just the individual" is clearly a value that brought her to medicine and provides energy and direction in her continuing journey in medicine.

STRATEGY 1: Find your personal statements

If you are like me, the application materials for educational programs are long gone. If you are more compulsive… or, let's say, thorough… you may be able to track down some education-related statements. Some people, I suppose, may have copies of college application essays or statements from graduate or professional schools. Schools certainly keep these materials for some period of time, as well.

You can also think more broadly about archival statements that touch on "purpose." Do you still have the cover letter and statement that you submitted for your current position? Have you applied for grant funding or research funding, when you have had occasion to describe why the project that you were proposing mattered to you?

If you are able to put your hands on any of this material, consider:

- What themes do you see in the values that were important to you at that point in your life? Why was it meaningful for you to pursue whatever step you were seeking at that point?
- Are these themes and values still important to you today? Have they been constant for you? Have they evolved?
- How does the work that you do now relate to the themes and values that you have identified?

STRATEGY 2

Write your own origin story

Cozy up with your laptop some evening, cabernet by your side (or fizzy water, if that is your choice beverage) and write about your own journey to doing what you now do. Suggestions:

- Just write. Start writing and keep going. The goal is not to produce articulate prose that would warm the heart of your high school English teacher, but to connect with the energy of some of the sentinel moments that have moved you in the directions that you have traveled.

- Focus on events, not theoretical concepts. When was a time when you first thought about being a nurse, or doctor, or massage therapist? What do you recall that may have set the stage for your being open to that first thought? When were some events that further refined your direction?

- Try to capture or re-create specific events with as much richness of experience as you can. You are the play-by-play guy and the color commentator at the same time. What did you see? What did you feel? What are some of the details that stand out in your memory? This level of description is inherently interesting and tends to engage the creative process in a way that stimulates additional recollections.

- If your journey includes epiphanies, fine. If your journey does not include epiphanies, fine. There are wonderful partner relationships that begin with love at first sight, and there are wonderful partner relationships where the acquaintance that people have one with another turns to fondness, turning to love and devotion. Some people have had a distinct sense of "calling" at a defined moment… if this is you, fine; if this is not you (it is not me), that is fine, too. Don't be deterred, in other words, if there is no single moment of glorious revelation, because journeys without these times are equally honorable and meaningful.

Write until you are done. You will know what that means. Pour some more fizzy water (one glass of cabernet is enough), or perhaps pack it up for a day or two, and then reflect on what this story reveals about purpose for you:

- Why do you think that you particularly recalled *these* events?
- Where is the energy that flows through the series of events that you have described? What are the themes in what has mattered to you?
- Was there some event among those that you have described that has a quality of sacredness to it? Was there a time when you felt like you were in a sacred space?
- How do you see the work that you now do as a part of this journey? When are the times in your work that you experience some of the same themes and energy that you find in your origin story?
- What might you do in your work… or in how you do your work… to allow it to more fully give expression to the themes of purpose that you have identified?

Personal mission

The second approach that supports the present awareness of purpose is personal mission.

Many companies have some articulation of *organizational* mission. Your organization is probably among them. Some mission statements are good. Some are not so good. The less compelling statements of mission tend to be written privately by a senior manager, duplicated, mounted on walls and promptly forgotten. The more vital and compelling statements of mission grow out of a process of conversation and discernment in a community of people working together.

Good statements of organizational mission:

- Describe the core purpose and values of the organization
- Can be remembered

- Provide energy and inspiration
- Help to chart directions

I was on sabbatical a number of years ago at the Seton Cove, which is a small spirituality center affiliated with the Seton Medical Center, a (then) Daughters of Charity hospital in Austin, Texas. Throughout the several campuses of the medical center hung tastefully artistic framed panels describing the "mission," "values" and "philosophy" of Seton Medical Center. The centerpiece of this display was the sentence, "We serve each person as a Christian would serve Christ himself."

This certainly describes a core value of the organization. It is memorable... striking, really, in the setting of the artistic display. I found it especially compelling, though, because it reminds staff of the sacred purpose of their work. The work is not just writing a script for hydrochlorothiazide, doing an MRI of someone's shoulder, setting somebody up for food stamps, or starting an IV... the work is serving people *as a follower of Christ would serve Christ himself.* Having the present awareness of this sacred value sets a profoundly different tone for our interactions with people than we would otherwise experience in exercising our technical skills alone.

Statements of organizational mission also help to chart direction. Another section of the Seton display of mission and values declares, "Our mission inspires us to care for and improve the health of those we serve with a special concern for the sick and the poor." Clearly, the shared understanding of this mission will help to chart direction. One can imagine some organizational initiatives that would fail the "special concern for the sick and the poor" criterion... promoting efficiency by treating Medicaid recipients in wards, rather than single or double rooms, for instance... and other organizational initiatives that would pass or honor this criterion.

Personal mission functions for us, as individuals, in the same way that statements of organizational mission function for groups of people working together. Like organizational statements, personal mission statements

- Describe the core purpose and values of the individual
- Can be remembered
- Provide energy and inspiration
- Help to chart directions

Consider some examples:

Having lost a child to a drunk driver, my mission is to relentlessly educate drivers about alcohol use, and to support other parents who have had this experience.

My mission is to help people to believe in themselves and to find some unique ways that they can make a difference.

My mission is to provide quality dental care, including care for some people who cannot pay for my services, and to treat my employees with dignity and respect.

I will pursue balance in my life, cherishing family and friends and also valuing my time alone, making a contribution in my workplace and also in my community, taking pride in how I relate to serious matters and also being able to laugh and be outrageous.

My service to this planet is to promote the flow of healing life energy through touch. In Massage, I will give the full attention of my soul to the people I see, allowing my own healing energy to flow through my hands and my spirit.

I think that all of these statements of personal mission speak to the four features I have suggested above. They describe core purpose, they are memorable, and you can easily imagine that they provide energy and direction. I personally prefer personal mission statements that are not career-specific as are the dental and massage examples, because I think that broader statements frame our approaches to work and to the rest of life, as well. The person in the example of "pursuing balance" can do this as a social worker and also as a husband, son, neighbor, community chorus member and in all of the other roles that he takes.

STRATEGY 3: Create a statement of personal mission

What would need to happen in order for you to feel "successful?" What will it look like when you are spiritually centered and devoting your energy and your heart to things that touch on your deepest values?

Experiment with developing a statement of personal mission as a way of focusing on... and directing you to... purpose.

Some guidelines: the three Cs of mission statements

- **Core.** A personal mission statement points the way to what you most want your life to be about. Your core purpose. What do you know from your own wisdom of experience about times when you really feel alive? When your intuition tells you that you are doing something that really matters?

  When are the times when you really feel spiritually renewed? When you are dis-spirited, what do you do that restores your soul? I had a friend many years ago who was a Catholic priest in a local parish. He said that whenever he was discouraged or demoralized, he would "visit somebody in the hospital." Never failed to cheer him up, he said. A good marker for core purpose.

- **Control.** The statement defines what you will do, or what you will be (we will consider this more in the next chapter). What you do is within your control; what other people do, or how other people receive you, is not within your control. Therefore, emphasize your own values and action, and go easy on statements of outcome that depend on other people and their choices.

"I will express and model kindness and caring with the children in my classes" is within a teacher's control. "I will make my second grade class the highest ranking in the Kansas City school system" is a laudable goal, but not a very good statement of core purpose.

Statements of mission often contain verbs that refer to ways that someone wants to relate to the world or to other people. Verbs like "encourage," "support," "challenge," "display," and "give expression."

- **Concise.** I have seen some statements of organizational and personal mission that run on for multiple paragraphs. Again, laudable, but not cool. If you are going to maintain the present awareness of purpose, the mission statement really should be a one- or two-liner, or, conceptually, should succinctly describe one or two ideas that you can keep in the forefront of your mind and recall with the same reliability as your social security number.

  People in the world of marketing refer to the "elevator speech." This describes a key idea in the time it takes to share an elevator journey with somebody between the 8th and 14th floors. (I don't think we have 14-story buildings in Maine, but I've heard tell...) *Why should I get on board with the building project?* (30 seconds). *Why should I support this research proposal?* (30 seconds). Same idea with personal mission statements... if it is incisive enough to describe to somebody in 30 seconds, it is probably focused and impactful enough that you can bear it in mind as you move through the day.

There are a number of helpful websites about developing statements of mission. Some good examples and resources for mission for organizations (in different sectors) and individuals, for instance are available at www.missionstatements.com.

Present awareness

The first challenge in "staying connected with purpose" is defining purpose in ways that matter to you. The second challenge is maintaining awareness of purpose. It does no good to chart the pathway to aliveness if you don't follow it.

The cardinal sin about mission in the organizational and management world is to define it and then forget it. Management literature talks about "alignment" with mission; making the awareness and understanding of mission so much a part of the daily life of the organization that the organizational values and purpose really drive the way that things happen. In our organization, for instance, the understanding of mission and values touches the recruitment process, the orientation of new employees, the evaluation of staff, and frequently can play a prominent role in planning meetings and retreats.

The goal is the same with values and purpose for individuals; to make the awareness and understanding of mission so much a part of daily life that our personal values and purpose really drive the way that we do things.

The idea of "present awareness" and "staying connected" with personal values and purpose permeates the several aspects of the personal arena of spiritual care. We will consider some specific approaches to "present awareness" as we explore qualities of character in the next chapter, and cultivating healing intention in Chapter 7.

For now, let me raise the issue and invite you to reflect on your own wisdom and approaches.

STRATEGY 4: Describe your own approach to "present awareness"

You have defined some elements of purpose in the settings of origin stories and personal mission. Reflect on your own experience with staying connected with purpose. How do you do this? When have there been times when you have been aware of purpose… core values... mission... and how did these times come about? Have you specifically engaged in practices that help you to stay connected with purpose. or do certain life events bring you to this awareness? What might you do that you think could enhance your day-to-day awareness of purpose and make this even more vitally a part of what you do?

SUMMARY

- Personal spiritual well-being (groundedness, wholeness, centeredness, aliveness) supports personal equanimity and helps us to provide creative, quality spiritual care.
- Staying connected with personal purpose is a key approach that promotes personal spiritual well-being.
- Two methodologies that direct us to personal purpose are origin stories and statements of personal mission.
- Both defining and cultivating day-to-day awareness of purpose are vital for us as providers of health and wellness care.

REFERENCES

1. Craigie FC, Jr., Hobbs RF. Exploring the organizational culture of exemplary community health center practices. Fam Med. 2004;36(10):733-738.
2. Jones LB, *The Path: Creating your Mission Statement for Work and for Life.* 1996. New York: Hyperion.

Chapter Six

The Moments of Your Life: Cultivate Qualities of Character

There is a vitality, a life force, an energy, a quickening that is translated through you into action, and because there is only one of you in all time, this expression is unique. And if you block it, it will never exist through any other medium and will be lost.

Martha Graham

What kind of person do you want to be? You may be defined by your profession, or your title, or… as we have discussed… by your purpose and mission, but you are also defined by your humanity. Your unique, "only one of you in all time" humanity. You express qualities of character, which you can really think of as sacred commitments to how you want to be living your life, in your day-to-day and moment-to-moment journey.

I remember the turning point for me, a couple of years ago. I was seeing a woman who would come in every two or three weeks complaining of some vaguely neurological problem… she didn't have feeling in her arms, or her legs would give out, or her field of vision was reduced, or she had weakness on one side or the other. She always checked out fine when I would examine her, but she kept insisting something was wrong that I was missing. No interest in behavioral consultation or counseling. Didn't want to go there at all. I referred her to a neurologist and she cancelled three scheduled appointments. I was really getting exasperated and was thinking of discharging her from my practice when it occurred to me… she can do what she wants to do or needs to do, and all I have to do is to be honest with her and be compassionate. I had always realized that compassion was one of my greatest strengths as a doctor, but it was really striking to realize that being honest and compassionate is enough with this person. I think I have certainly felt better and I think she has as well since then.

In this chapter, we will consider the importance, within the personal arena of spiritual care, of cultivating qualities of character. Qualities like the compassion of this physician, or inquisitiveness, creativity, love of learning, or joy… represent not so much "mission" or "purpose" as I have described, but qualities that define the kind of person that you wish to be.

Qualities of character are important for three reasons. First, the cultivation of qualities of character that are particularly and personally significant for each of us ***promotes our own spiritual well-being***. If you value kindness, then you will be most alive spiritually as you are kind. If you value gratitude, then you will be most alive when you are grateful. If you value perseverance, then you will be most alive as you are resolutely making your way through challenges.

Second, our cultivation of qualities of character ***helps us to provide good health and wellness care.*** Whatever it is that you most cherish about how you wish to live your life, it is the connection and expression of those qualities that help you to be centered and grounded. When you are centered and grounded, your presence with people… and the spirit that you bring to your work… will be palpably different from when you are not. When you are really present with people, you are already providing good, foundational, spiritual care.

The third reason is that the expression of qualities of character *puts distinct energy out into the world, and this energy spreads and endures.* When you are joyful or forthright or charitable, you put distinct energy out there and this energy spreads and endures.

A number of years ago, my wife and I visited the Penn Center in South Carolina. Located on St. Helena Island, the Penn Center was of one of the country's first schools for freed slaves. It was founded in 1862 when Union forces captured the South Carolina Sea Islands and it remained in Union hands for the remainder of the Civil War. In its very early days, the center recruited two young women from Philadelphia who came to the school as teachers and lived among and educated former Sea Island slaves for the next forty years.

Today, the Penn Center remains a significant African American historical and cultural institution. In the museum that traces the history of the center, there is a striking photograph that was taken shortly after the founding of the school. It shows a group of people gathered around the doorway of a former slave cabin. In the foreground is one of the teachers, back to the camera. She faces a former slave woman and her daughter who have the kind of blank expressions that were typical of mid-nineteenth century photography. In the doorway is a young boy of seven or eight, presumably the son of the woman, who has the most radiant smile. His expression is one of delight, perhaps with a little mischief. My guess is that the teacher has just said something to tease the boy, or maybe they had teased each other.

What is striking to me about the photograph is the enduring energy of that moment. In the middle of a long and terrible war, here is a fleeting moment of grace, lasting perhaps a second, perhaps a few seconds. The energy in that moment in that relationship in 1862, perhaps long forgotten by the participants, didn't die there. It endures, touching a middle-aged white couple walking by over 140 years later.

POSITIVE PSYCHOLOGY

The importance of qualities of character for well-being has been developed extensively in the positive psychology movement. Growing out of the mid-twentieth century work on mental well-being exemplified by Carl Rogers and Abraham Maslow, positive psychology concerns itself with "positive emotions, positive character traits and enabling institutions."[1] Rather than focusing on mental distress, positive psychology focuses on the qualities and approaches that make life worth living and that contribute to happiness, satisfaction and fulfillment.

According to positive psychology, both historical tradition and contemporary research point to three principal orientations to happiness and well-being.[2] The first, rooted in the ancient doctrine of hedonism, emphasizes the pursuit of **pleasurable experiences and the minimization of pain**. As I write this, with the January temperature in Maine hovering near zero, the example of warm southern vacations comes to mind.

The second, referred to as **"engagement,"** emphasizes people's relationships with activities and pursuits that absorb our attention over substantial periods of time. Many of us, for instance, have a Great Aunt who is devoted to genealogy and who spends countless hours pouring over transatlantic ship logs and American census data. In the modern literature, the orientation of engagement is represented best by the work on states of "flow."[3]

The third orientation to happiness and well-being emphasizes the pursuit of **meaning**. This orientation has its roots in the Aristotelian idea of eudaimonia; "striving toward excellence based on one's unique potential." A cultural assumption of Aristotle's day was that people (mainly, property-owning men) were all endowed with an individual *daimon*, or a kind of personal spirit, with unique in-dwelling dispositions and talents. Writing in the Fourth Century BCE, Aristotle argued that human fulfillment comes from people being faithful to their individual daimons, in ways that would reveal the best that is within them.

In modern language, we might speak of people giving expression to their unique talents, passions and character. Someone who is particularly oriented to a spirit of charity, for instance, would pursue meaning and fulfillment by being charitable. He or she might do this in more organized ways, like setting up a soup kitchen, or less formal and organized ways, like reacting to mistreatment with patience and grace.

Research suggests that personal well-being and life satisfaction are associated with all three of these orientations, with engagement and meaning having stronger influences than pleasure.[4] In addition to quality of life benefits, moreover, there are data that eudaimonia… life marked by high levels of purpose and growth… is associated with a variety of positive biological markers in areas such as cardiovascular, neuroendocrine and immune function.[5, 6]

Character Strengths and Virtues

The sentinel work on qualities of character comes from a multi-year, cross-cultural research project chaired by Drs. Martin Seligman from the University of Pennsylvania and Christopher Peterson from the University of Michigan. Seligman had originally been invited to take part in conversations about developing programs to improve the character of young people. After a day of dialogue with other experts in youth development, there was a shared recognition that the field lacked a dependable system for defining character, and that a classification system was necessary in order to direct and evaluate whatever programs that the group might develop. Seligman took on the task of developing such a system of classification, recruiting Peterson and a number of other colleagues.

Together, they launched upon a landmark study of wisdom about character across cultures and across the span of human history.[7] The question was whether there were universal beliefs about virtue and character that would be consistent across the broad range of traditions that they reviewed. They mapped out a campaign to review documents and writings from all of the major religious and philosophical traditions... ancient Greece and Rome, Confucius, Buddha, Jewish and Christian sources, Lao-Tze, the Koran, Charlemagne, and relatively modern figures from Benjamin Franklin to Sir John Templeton. They even included an admirable and, I'm sure, intriguing anthropological examination of assumptions about virtue and character in contemporary iconic cultural sources such as Hallmark greeting cards, bumper stickers, popular song lyrics, Saturday Evening Post covers and Pokémon characters.

Growing out of this body of research, Seligman and colleagues did indeed discover that there are nearly-universal themes about human virtue. They organized their findings into six categories of virtue, as you see in the table.

Classification of 6 Virtues and 24 Character Strengths (Peterson & Seligman, 2004)

Virtue and strength	Definition
1. Wisdom and knowledge	Cognitive strengths that entail the acquisition and use of knowledge
Creativity	Thinking of novel and productive ways to do things
Curiosity	Taking an interest in all of ongoing experience
Open-mindedness	Thinking things through and examining them from all sides
Love of learning	Mastering new skills, topics, and bodies of knowledge
Perspective	Being able to provide wise counsel to others
2. Courage	Emotional strengths that involve the exercise of will to accomplish goals in the face of opposition, external or internal
Authenticity	Speaking the truth and presenting oneself in a genuine way
Bravery	Not shrinking from threat, challenge, difficulty, or pain
Persistence	Finishing what one starts
Zest	Approaching life with excitement and energy
3. Humanity	Interpersonal strengths that involve "tending and befriending" others
Kindness	Doing favors and good deeds for others
Love	Valuing close relations with others
Social intelligence	Being aware of the motives and feelings of self and others
4. Justice	Civic strengths that underlie healthy community life
Fairness	Treating all people the same according to notions of fairness and justice
Leadership	Organizing group activities and seeing that they happen
Teamwork	Working well as member of a group or team
5. Temperance	Strengths that protect against excess
Forgiveness	Forgiving those who have done wrong
Modesty	Letting one's accomplishments speak for themselves
Prudence	Being careful about one's choices; not saying or doing things that might later be regretted
Self-regulation	Regulating what one feels and does
6. Transcendence	Strengths that forge connections to the larger universe and provide meaning
Appreciation of beauty and excellence	Noticing and appreciating beauty, excellence, and/or skilled performance in all domains of life
Gratitude	Being aware of and thankful for the good things that happen
Hope	Expecting the best and working to achieve it
Humor	Liking to laugh and tease; bringing smiles to other people
Religiousness	Having coherent beliefs about the higher purpose and meaning of life

from: Peterson C, Seligman M. *Character Strengths and Virtues: A Handbook and Classification.* New York: American Psychological Association/Oxford University Press; 2004. Reprinted with permission.

Wisdom and knowledge, courage, humanity, justice, temperance, and transcendence, in other words, are core characteristics that are valued across time and cultures by moral philosophers and religious thinkers (not to mention singer-songwriters, cartoon designers and entrepreneurial pundits).

For each of these categories of virtue, the Seligman research describes three or more corresponding strengths of character. Strengths of character are pathways to the virtues... routes to cultivating and displaying the virtues. The virtue of "humanity," therefore, is approached and displayed by kindness, love, and social intelligence.

It is at this level of strengths of character that the system has practical implications. While the six virtues are universally esteemed across cultures, the twenty-four strengths of character vary considerably in their personal importance among individuals. It is as if people are hard-wired for some of the strengths of character to be more or less important. You and I may both hold the virtues in equal esteem, but you may be hard-wired to the expression of creativity and curiosity, while I may be hard-wired to the expression of different character strengths... say, gratitude and hope. In the positive psychology framework, the two or three strongest hard-wired strengths of character are referred to as our "signature strengths."

The practical application of this program of research is that happiness and fulfillment are very significantly related to the expression of signature strengths. If your signature strengths are creativity and curiosity, then your happiness and fulfillment will be significantly related to the extent to which you give expression to these strengths by some creative pursuits and by inquisitiveness about the way things work. This relationship of signature strengths and well-being is observed for all of the strengths, but it particularly robust for strengths "of the heart;" zest, gratitude, hope, and love.

I find this to be a very helpful framework, and I speak about it frequently with patients and with clinicians. Strengths of character are important for the reasons we have considered... promoting spiritual well-being, enhancing clinical care, and putting out energy that endures… and also because our expression of strengths of character is under our control. This powerful force for well-being and healing is under our discretionary control. You may not be able to control how many phone calls you need to return, or what services the managed care company denies, or whether or not patients choose to use passion flower tea as you have suggested, but you can always choose whether to be kind, or open-minded, or persistent, or grateful.

DISCOVERING QUALITIES OF CHARACTER

Generally, the literature about strengths of character suggests that we focus our attention on identifying and cultivating signature strengths… those strengths of character that are hard-wired to be individually important to us. I think this is a good approach, with the caveat that it can also be meaningful to identify and experiment with qualities of character that are not signature strengths. If "gratitude" and "hope" are signature strengths for me, then I will nurture my own spiritual well-being by cultivating and expressing these strengths… being grateful, expressing thanks, recognizing blessings, and expecting and working toward good outcomes. At the same time, if my less-strong personal strengths of character are "authenticity" and "bravery," then it can be meaningful for me to look for ways to give expression to these qualities… expressing honest feelings or unpopular opinions, for instance.

A word about language, by the way. The Peterson/Seligman framework is rooted in extensive research, and the use of their words to describe qualities of character has some empirical basis and intuitive appeal. I wouldn't assume that this language has a corner on the market for thinking about qualities of character, though. As I will suggest in the next section about clinical approaches, I think that there is often great value in organizing conversations around language that comes from the people we work with. A patient last week, for instance, says that his goal is to be "at peace." This is not the customary language of health care, but it is meaningful for him. Rather than substitute my own language ("Hm, do you mean that you would like to have an enhanced sense of self-efficacy?"), I would usually work with the words and concepts that have personal meaning to him, and where he has some ownership of the language.

Same idea with qualities of character. We can certainly use the Peterson/Seligman language, but we can also invent our own. I worked with a nurse, for instance, who wished to be more "charitable" in her feelings and approaches to patients and colleagues. "Charity" does not appear among the 24 strengths of character in the framework I have described (it is perhaps related to "kindness" or "forgiveness"), but it is a perfectly appropriate and honorable focus of her attention.

There are three principal approaches to discovering signature strengths and other qualities of character that have personal meaning for us.

Inventories

Questionnaires that specifically assess the strengths of character from the Peterson/Seligman research are available in paper and electronic formats. Seligman has written a popular-press book, *Authentic Happiness,*[8] that nicely summarizes the character strengths and values projects and has a number of self-tests, including the assessment of character strengths. I recommend this to many people. As I write this, you can get 87 new and used copies from $6.59 from amazon.com. Always a bargain.

A more thorough and definitive version of the character strengths inventory (the form that has been used in the main body of research) is available online at www.authentichappiness.org. This website is Seligman's University of Pennsylvania portal for public access to information and resources about a variety of positive psychology projects. You register (for free) and receive unlimited access to the strengths inventory and some fascinating related material for

self-assessment of happiness, gratitude, forgiveness, work-life satisfaction, compassionate love, and other related qualities.

The character strengths inventory is the "VIA Signature
Strengths Questionnaire." This 240-question inventory gives you
feedback about the rank order of your self-assessed strengths of
each of the 24 qualities of character. A brief version of this inventory, appropriately called the "Brief Strengths Test," gives you
feedback about your percentile rank for each of the character
strengths among web users and fellow test-takers in your gender,
age group, educational cohort, occupational group and zip code.
My personal experience, by the way, is that my percentile rankings
for my zip code almost always were higher (my character strengths
compared to my neighbors) than my percentile rankings among
web users overall (my character strengths compared to my Internet
compatriots). I must live in a rough town.

There are a large number of other resources out there which,
similarly, help to focus the exploration of personal values and
qualities of character. Among them, I also frequently recommend
a great "sortable" list of personal values from Dr. William Miller at
the University of New Mexico (http://motivationalinterview.org/
library/valuescardsort.pdf). You may recognize Miller as one of
the developers of the motivational interviewing paradigm; he has
had a remarkably creative and prolific career with substance abuse
treatment and spirituality, among other areas.

Conversation and feedback

Ask your partner. Ask your colleagues. Ask your friends. If you
are daring and stout of heart, ask your children. What do they
see in you that they admire? What qualities of character come to
mind when they think about their observations and relationships
with you? What do they think you uniquely contribute to the way
things run around here?

A hospital middle manager recounts performance feedback:

*It was touching, actually. My supervisor said that everyone knew
I could be loud and boisterous and sometimes say pretty outlandish
things… and we talked about maybe I could tone that down a notch…
but she said that it was always absolutely clear that I respected the
people I work with and honor their opinions and choices. I really do,
and it was nice to hear that she sees this in me.*

Your own reflection

Finally, you can just create some time and space to think about it
yourself. Consider:

- What do you particularly take pride in with regard to how
  you try to live your life day to day? What kind of person do
  you try to be?
- When have there been times when you have really felt positive
  about what you were doing? What memorable events do
  you recall that felt good emotionally and spiritually? What
  qualities of character are visible in these events?
- How do you want to be living and handling the challenging
  situations that come your way?
- When are the times when you feel like you are really connecting with a patient, friend or family member?
- When are the times when your energy or spirit brings a little
  light or goodness into the world?
- What does it mean to you to be a healer and when are the
  times when you are really giving life to your calling or vocation?
- Recalling Howard Thurman's comment, what does it mean
  to you to "come alive" and when/how does this happen?
- If you were planning to move to Bozeman, Montana, and had a
  going-away gathering of your friends and associates, what would
  you hope and expect they would say about you? (Bozeman seems
  like a good example of a far-removed destination for someone
  who lives in Maine; if you happen to live in Montana, you can

substitute "Caribou, Maine.") This is, by the way, a question that is related to the 1970s "legacy" exercise from the human potential movement of imagining yourself at your funeral, except without so much a spirit of finality. In either case, the point of self-reflection is to envision the particular words of affection and admiration from people who care about you.

STRATEGY 5: Identify your own signature strengths of character

Use any of the methodologies and approaches we have considered above to discover or focus your attention on qualities of character that are particularly meaningful for you.

An additional approach you might consider is to reflect on "you at your best." This is another particular exercise that grows out of the Peterson/Seligman work, and I speak about this frequently. The task is to recall some specific day-to-day event that shows "you at your best." It is not so much oriented to formal or publicly-visible accomplishments ("chairing the staffing study committee," "getting the employee of the month award… with the premium parking space") as it is oriented to day-to-day expressions of how you live your life.

An example I sometimes describe to groups:

I play a lot of basketball and typically find myself playing with people who are years or decades younger. At my age, this is pretty much the way it goes. I was playing pickup basketball some time ago at the local YMCA… "pickup" meaning that people forms teams just in order of arrival… and had two people I knew and two people I didn't know on my team. The two people I didn't know were in their late teens and apparently came together. It was immediately apparent that they didn't have much of a clue about playing the game. They were not quite on top of some basic basketball rules, such as when you have to dribble when you move around the court, and they put up shots that missed the rim and the backboard completely.

One of the two people I knew, Ted, was a young man in his mid twenties who finished school in the last couple of years and comes when his work schedule allows. I need to mention, here, that the culture of men's basketball generally is that when people show up who don't contribute much to the game... let alone people who are so lost at sea... the manly response is to ignore them and play as though they were not there. I tried, myself, to be encouraging of our younger teammates, and I was particularity surprised and struck by how Ted treated them. He passed the ball to them. He resisted the temptation to roll his eyes. He said words of encouragement; "Go ahead, brother, shoot the ball."

When the game was over, I went up to Ted and told him how impressed I was at how he had treated the two younger guys. In the fine art of manly interchange, he nodded without saying anything, but it was clear that he knew what I meant.

This is an example that comes to mind when I think of me at my best; trying to be fair and inclusive of other people and being encouraging and affirming when I see people behaving in kind and generous ways. It is a day-to-day example that has nothing to do with academic rank or publications, but it captures something of the person that I try to be.

So... identify your own strengths of character. And tell somebody about it.

WORKING WITH QUALITIES OF CHARACTER

You have determined some patterns in your qualities of character that are relatively prominent and meaningful for you, and perhaps some that are less so. Now what?

Present awareness

My primary suggestion for working with qualities of character is to hold them in your awareness. In the last chapter, I used the phrase, "maintaining present awareness." Even without deliberately setting out to change anything, it can often be meaningful just to be aware of things that we value. The rationale is that *what we focus our attention and hearts on tends to grow.* All of us wrestle daily with the imperative to focus our attention and hearts on things that don't matter, things that we don't value, and what is wrong in ourselves and the world. The spiritually-affirming process is the opposite; focusing attention and heart on what matters. If you value open-mindedness, fairness, social intelligence, or gratitude… maintain these qualities in your awareness. Keep them in front of you.

Some approaches:

- **Journaling**. Give voice to what you see and experience about the qualities of character that you value. Pick a time daily to reflect and write. I will speak more about journaling in a clinical context, but I can say here that there is some excellent literature about the value of daily journaling in a format of writing (with minimal editing) and then reflecting about what you can learn from what you have written. Dr. James Pennebaker from the University of Texas has worked extensively with this process.[9-11]

- **Periodic check-in**. Pick a couple of times during the day to check in about a particular value or quality of character. "How has 'hope' come up for me this morning?" "When have I experienced 'zest' this afternoon?" "What opportunities might I have to give expression to 'bravery' in the next couple of days?" For some people, times to hold values in awareness are built into the rhythm of their days… as in private devotions, meditation, or grace before meals. For other people, it may be a little more catch-as-catch-can.

- **Retreats**. Many spiritual and religious traditions encourage periodic retreats. Many communities have retreat centers that offer peaceful settings for contemplation and often, humble overnight accommodations. When I was on sabbatical at Fuller Theological Seminary many years ago, I would frequently spend a few minutes during the day in a marvelous meditation garden. In the midst of the traffic and bustle of metropolitan Los Angeles, the garden had been designed with a several-foot-high wall of continually cascading water, which served to attenuate sound and to provide a visual focal point. Similarly, I suspect that you have peaceful and sacred places that are meaningful for you.

- **Community**. "How am I doing with forgiveness?" is not the kind of conversation that most of us have very frequently. However, it can be powerful to share one's journey with a community of other people with whom this kind of conversation is possible. For many years before we all went our separate ways, I got together weekly for an hour... a very early hour... with three other men who were also involved in spiritual and psychological care. This provided a rich opportunity for us to celebrate the joys of our lives, to support one another in the challenging times, and to be accountable for the directions in which we wanted to be going.

With these or other approaches, you may maintain awareness of qualities of character that matter to you. Consider how they are part of your daily life. Reflect on what flows well. What gets in the way? What differences do you see yourself making in your life and relationships as you express these values? What are you learning from this exercise and where do you see yourself going from here?

Expressing character qualities in new ways

In the present awareness and observation of qualities of character, things may change. If, indeed, focusing attention and heart on things that matter to us causes them to grow, then we would expect strengths of character to grow with awareness.

In addition to the unforeseen changes that may arise out of this awareness, you can be intentional about cultivating particular qualities of character. One of the stock exercises from the positive psychology movement is to explore how you might express signature strengths in new ways. Perhaps a personally-meaningful character strength for you is "curiosity." Perhaps this most often takes shape for you in the context of active inquiry in your field of expertise. "What do we know about integrative medicine treatments for irritable bowel syndrome?" "How much of the effectiveness of antidepressants is attributable to expectancy effects?" "Is passion flower more effective as a tincture or as a tea?"

How, then, might you express curiosity in ways that are new for you? You could write poetry, with a curious spirit about what you may stand to learn or discover. You could write music, learning about the mathematics and the soul of tonal relationships. You could talk in an earnestly inquisitive way to a Republican if you are a Democrat, or a Democrat if you are a Republican. You could pay close attention to the flow of conversation in team planning meetings, and see whether there are totally novel and creative approaches that no one else is considering.

Experiment with less prominent strengths

If your inventory results, your conversations, or your intuition suggest particular qualities of character that are not prominent for you, try them out. If "bravery" is low on your list, be brave. If "modesty" is low on your list, be modest. If "forgiveness" is low on your list, forgive.

I have never been particularly engaged with the Myers-Briggs paradigm,[12] but I have appreciated the point that MBTI folks make about more-preferred and less-preferred styles. For each of the pairings of ways of relating to the world (introversion/extraversion, sensing/intuition, thinking/feeling, judging/perceiving), people are most comfortable and capable operating from their preferred styles, and people grow most from operating from their less preferred styles.

STRATEGY 6
Nurture your own character

Choose one among the approaches to "working with qualities of character" that appeals to you. Maintain awareness of your signature strengths. Express them in new ways. Experiment with qualities of character that are less familiar and comfortable for you.

SUMMARY

- Cultivating our own qualities of character is a vital element in providing good spiritual care.
- Cultivating our own qualities of character is important because
  - It promotes our own spiritual well-being.
  - It helps us to provide good health and wellness care.
  - It puts positive energy out into the world, and this energy spreads and endures.
- Positive Psychology, with its empirically-based framework of character strengths and virtues, provides a rich set of resources for cultivating meaningful personal qualities.
- We discover personally-meaningful qualities of character with
  - inventories
  - conversation and feedback
  - personal reflection
- We nurture and grow qualities of character by holding them in awareness and by exploring ways to give expression to them in our daily lives and relationships.

REFERENCES

1. Seligman M, Steen T, Park N, Peterson C. Positive psychology progress: Empirical validation of interventions. *Am Psychol.* 2005;60(5):410-421.
2. Peterson C, Ruch W, Beerman U, Park N, Seligman M. Strengths of character, orientations to happiness, and life satisfaction. *J Pos Psych.* 2007;2(3):149-156.

3. Csikszentmihalyi M. *Flow: The Psychology of Optimal Experience.* New York: Harper & Row; 1990.

4. Peterson C, Park N, Seligman M. Orientations to happiness and life satisfaction: The full life versus the empty life. *J Happ Stud.* 2005;6:25-41.

5. Ryff C, Singer B, Dienberg Love G. Positive health: Connecting well-being with biology. *Philos Trans R Soc Lond B Biol Sci.* 2004;359(1449):1383-1394.

6. Friedman E, Hayney M, Love G, Singer B, Ryff C. Plasma interleukin-6 and soluble IL-6 receptors are associated with psychological well-being in aging women. *Health Psychol.* 2007;26(3):305-313.

7. Peterson C, Seligman M. *Character Strengths and Virtues: A Handbook and Classification.* New York: American Psychological Association/ Oxford University Press; 2004.

8. Seligman M. *Authentic Happiness.* New York: Free Press; 2002.

9. Pennebaker J. *Opening Up: The Healing Power of Expressing Emotions.* New York: Guilford; 1997.

10. Pennebaker J. The effects of traumatic disclosure on physical and mental health: The values of writing and talking about upsetting events. *Int J Emerg Ment Health.* 1999;1(1):9-18.

11. Pennebaker J. Forming a story: The health benefits of narrative. *J Clin Psych.* 1999;55(10):1243-1254.

12. Kiersey D, Bates M. *Please Understand Me: Character and Temperament Types.* Del Mar, CA: Prometheus Nemesis Book Company; 1984.

Chapter Seven

Ground Yourself in Healing Intention and Presence

Your vision will become clear only when you look into your own heart.
Who looks outside, dreams; who looks inside, awakens.

Carl Jung

In exploring the personal arena of spiritual care, we have considered the importance of staying connected with purpose and of cultivating strengths of character. Equally important is our intention to be healers in people's lives and the expression of that intention, which is to be fully present with people.

Years ago I developed a ritual which I follow faithfully every day. Before I go into an exam room to see a patient, I pause for a few seconds outside, feet flat of the floor, and remind myself why I want to be there with the person I am about to see. For me, it helps me let go of whatever else is going on and helps me to be able to look people in the eye and to really be there with them. It helps me to be a better doctor.

As Jung says, it starts in our own hearts… the intention to be here, now, with this person. Our healing intention helps us to be fully present, and supports the realization of purpose, and creates an environment where our strengths of character come to life.

INTENTION AND PRESENCE

It is a package deal, intention and presence. Clarity of intention helps us to be present with people, and it is hard to be present to people without clarity of intention.

Explorations of intention and presence in clinical or healing settings have recognized this connection. Dr. Norman Shealey, neurosurgeon and founding president of the American Holistic Medical Association, has studied prominent, exemplary healers around the world. He finds two recurring qualities.[1] First, exemplary healers hold "intention to heal." Often entering still and prayerful states, these master healers visualize or anticipate the healing of sick people, "allowing intention to be the vehicle through which the power of healing can move." Second, they manifest and relate to people with what Shealey calls "calm emotional states... such as love, peace, compassion and tranquility." Even if there may be turmoil elsewhere in their personal lives, their visible and palpable presence in the setting of healing is one of compassion and serenity.

Similarly, Dr. David Rakel, author/editor of the landmark textbook, *Integrative Medicine, 2nd Ed.* (Saunders, 2007), comments,

Being fully present with positive intention to another human being is perceived by those we are with and enhances the healing effects of the encounters. It is difficult to truly connect with intention until we have explored our own inner nature. Patient care starts with ourselves. As this connection grows, our ability to sit fully with another suffering human will be enhanced... this growth brings forth foundations in healing that include positive expectation, hope, faith, and unconditional positive regard. (p. 16)

Intention and compassionate presence are woven together. We can, however, look at some perspectives on intention and presence separately.

Mechanisms and effects of healing intention

Intention can have indirect effects or direct effects. Indirect effects occur when a state of healing intention influences some other variable or quality which, in turn, has an effect on outcomes. In the relationship between intention and presence, intention would have an indirect effect on health outcomes insofar as intention helps clinicians to be more compassionate, more fully present, and more open to intuitive approaches... and it is compassion, presence and intuition that have healing effects. This is profoundly important, but I also suspect that it is fairly incontrovertible at this point. Good news, old news.

No less important, and really quite intriguing, is the possibility of direct effects of intention... that intention can have measurable outcomes without the mediating effects of personal contact. Praying for someone without being present and without their awareness, for instance, would be a setting in which there could be direct effects of intention.

There is growing anecdotal and scientific literature on direct effects of intention. The word "intention" sometimes accompanies this literature, and sometimes there are other frameworks and linguistic anchors such as "consciousness," "energy," "synchronicity," "distant," and "nonlocal," among others. Consider the following:

Laboratory studies reveal a variety of effects of intention with nonliving and living systems. Distant intention affects the rolls of dice, over many thousands of trials, to a small but statistically significant extent. Distant intention has been shown both to impede and stimulate significantly the growth of cultures of bacteria[2] and to influence the directions of bacterial mutations.[3] With mammals, non-contact healing intent cured mice of transplanted mammary adenocarcinoma to a significantly greater extent than controls.[4]

Laboratory studies with humans has shown that positive mental intent influences EEG patterns and formation of images in distant receivers when there is no physical connection by which such effects would be explained. Summarizing such studies, Mehl-Madrona comments, "These and other experiments provide significant evidence that identifiable and consistent electrical signals occur in the brain of one person when a second person, especially if he or she is closely related or emotionally linked, is either meditating, or provided with sensory stimulation, or attempts to communicate with the subject intentionally."[5]

Clinical studies of remote intercessory prayer and other distant healing have shown beneficial effects with patients with cardiac disease[6, 7] and AIDS.[8] The sentinel study of such effects examined distant prayer with 393 subjects in a coronary care unit.[7] Subjects in the experimental group, the recipients of prayer (none of whom were aware they were being prayed for), showed a series of clinical outcome advantages over a non-prayed-for control group. To statistically significant degrees, experimental subjects required less mechanical ventilation and less antibiotics and diuretics, had fewer cardiopulmonary arrests and episodes of pneumonia, and had lower "severity scores" reflecting their overall hospital course.

Recent meta-analytic reviews of distant healing in clinical settings, by the way, show some mixed results (with definitive conclusions being elusive because of methodological variations), but enough promising effects to warrant continued examination.[9, 10] Astin and colleagues, for instance, reviewed 23 trials of distant healing (primarily prayer and non-contact therapeutic touch) and found that 57% showed statistically significant treatment effects.[9]

Apart from published research, the case for direct effects of intention and nonlocal outcomes is compelling. A patient of mine a couple of years ago had the experience of awakening at night hearing her grandmother, in another state, telling her gently that she was loved and that "it would be all right." In the morning, she called her sister in the Upper Midwest (also at a distance from the grandmother), who had had the same experience. Together, they called the local family who supervised the grandmother and learned that she had passed away.

In a less dramatic but comparably compelling way, we have had the experience in our family when one of us (my wife and I and our three grown children) calls another of us… at an irregular and completely unpredictable time… and finds that the recipient of the call was reaching for the phone to call the caller. This has happened countless times, sometimes with the uncanny precision that the recipient picks up the phone in that instant when the connection is made before the phone actually rings.

Similarly, my wife and I have many times been driving long distances together (which is what you do when you live in a large, rural state), not talking for ten or fifteen minutes (Mainers are laconic, you understand), and one of us will make some comment… to which the other person responds, "That's *just* what I was thinking about."

We have come to consider such experiences between and among us completely normal, and it has been interesting and affirming to hear from friends and colleagues that many other people seem to experience these events, as well.

Compassionate presence

An EMT relates,

We responded to a neat and tidy trailer on the edge of town… a presumed heart attack. We found a little old man… thin, I'll bet he didn't weigh a hundred pounds, and his wife. He was clearly in distress and we put him in the ambulance for the 15 minute ride. He spoke French and I don't, so we really couldn't talk, but I could sense that he was really afraid… I guessed for himself and for his wife who he's probably been married to forever. I just held his hand and even though he was really in pain, he squeezed my hand tight and wouldn't take his eyes off of my eyes. I felt a real warmth and connection between us, even without words. It seemed to me that the fear in his eyes gave way to more of a feeling of peacefulness, maybe gratitude. I could tell that my being there like that for him meant something to him, and I guess that look of fear changing to peacefulness has stayed with me and means something to me. He died the next day.

One can look specifically at compassionate presence, as well. The parameters and benefits of presence are abundantly documented in the literature of nursing, medicine, behavioral health and complementary and integrative medicine.

Psychotherapy outcome research, for instance, consistently shows that "presence" or "relationship" contributes more toward therapeutic outcomes than does the particular method of therapy. Reviewing 40 years of outcome research, for instance, Hubble, Duncan and Miller[11] report that the largest contributor to therapeutic outcome is "extratherapeutic effects and client factors." Your lonely 28 year old patient with the DSM diagnosis of major depression meets a loving and attentive partner and his depression remits. Beyond such effects, the largest contributing factor to the remaining variance in outcome is "alliance factors," indicating whether there is a present, respectful and collaborative relationship between clinician and client. These factors are almost eight times more important, in terms of their statistical contribution to outcomes, than are factors related to model or technique.

In the *family systems literature,* Edwin Friedman has written persuasively about the importance of a "non-anxious presence" in families and organizational settings.[12] A non-anxious presence is both "present" and "non-anxious," and the ability to be fully present with a spirit of measured calm can significantly change the energy of emotionally charged situations.

In *health care,* there have been a number of studies, conceptual cousins to the Shealey research on exemplary healers, that have deconstructed healing relationships or presence. A 2008 study from Vanderbilt, for instance, identified 50 physicians from 3 states who were regarded by their professional peers as having exemplary relationships with their patients.[13] Interviews were conducted with these physicians, centering on the questions, "How do you go about establishing and maintaining healing relationships with your patients," and "What concrete things do you do to bring this about?" Using a qualitative content analysis methodology, the authors identified eight themes. These themes represent some specific constituent parts of healing presence… "Take time and listen," "Be open," "Find something to like and love…" that you can envision would make for the kinds of relationships that resulted in these physicians being nominated as experts.

Similarly, Laidlaw and colleagues looked at qualities that distinguished another group of physicians who had been identified as "exemplary communicators" from those who had not.[14] Their research approach involved actual behavioral samples and observations, having these physicians participate in videotaped OSCEs ("objective structured clinical examinations," a methodological hot ticket in the world of medical education) focusing on adolescent sexual health issues. With a quantitative analysis of several measures, they found that three skills differentiated the exemplary communicators from their less distinguished peers; "empathy," "non-judgment," and "self-reflection."

If you are particularly interested in the issue of healing presence and why it is important, by the way, I can suggest an especially thorough and scholarly review from the University of Arizona.[15] McDonough-Means and colleagues review existing literature, present an integrated systemic model about healing presence, and propose an articulate program of directions for research.

There is, in other words, substantial empirical literature from several angles about the effects of compassionate presence in human relationships. As a practical matter, the compassionate presence of clinicians is profoundly important because it creates an honoring and safe space for patients to be forthcoming about their lives, their fears, and their values. A few months ago, I saw a man who had had a somewhat wayward youth and had been packed away to a reform school for boys in his early teen years. While there, he was sexually abused by a guard for a couple of years. Now in his sixties, he had held this information secret (apart from his wife) for his entire life, until he decided that he had to make peace with this part of his past. He made clinic appointments and disclosed this information to his primary care physician (who is a particularly compassionate person) and to me. He had had some contact with both of us before and commented that it was extraordinarily difficult to face and disclose this history, but that he knew he would be "safe" speaking with both of us.

Intention, presence and intuition

We have considered earlier the proposition that personal well-being of clinicians is important... among other reasons... because it helps us to be more open to the flow and energy of intuition. The same idea pertains to the package combination of intention and presence; when we are intentional and focused with people, we are also more open to intuition. We are better able to be creative, or open to a creative spirit, in exploring patients' stories and in suggesting some new directions.

Dr. Wayne Dyer, psychologist and widely-published author about personal growth, expands on this idea in his 2004 book, *The Power of Intention.*[16] In his use of the word "intention," he means an omnipresent force in the universe... an "energy field of intent," "Spirit working through you," "inspiration or in-spiriting," and "infinite potential." This perspective on "intention" is really very much akin to what I am calling "flow and energy of intuition" and "creative spirit." Different spiritual traditions may also associate this with language like "God," "the Universe" and "Higher Power." The idea, essentially, is that there is wisdom out there, to which we are more fully open when we are spiritually present and grounded. In Dyer's framework, he describes a number of perspectives and approaches that help us to connect to this intention, such as being creative, being kind, being loving, and appreciating beauty.

Consider another clinical example of intention, presence and intuition in clinical care. A young divorced woman, who had taken leave of a teaching job because of "a breakdown," had been working with me in pulling her life together and charting some directions when she received word from another state that her ex-husband's mother had died. There was no love lost for her ex-husband and she was really quite intimidated by much of his family but she had had a very fond relationship with her mother-in-law. She debated whether to go to the funeral. We considered this together. The usual counseling approaches ("What would be the worst that could happen? "How would you handle it if...?) did not particularly help her to become more settled about a decision. It occurred to me to ask her, "Let's look at this from another direction... if you go there, what do you think that you would bring... that your presence there would bring... that would be unique to you, that no one else would offer?" She paused and thought about this. She said, "Maybe I can go there and just be who I am and just show them that I loved Betty... and that's all I have to do." She did go, and reported when she returned that it had been a rich and growing experience for her.

I give this example not because it attests to Dr. Craigie's skill as a therapist, but because the impetus for asking the questions that turned out to be pivotal was a matter of inspiration. As with the oncology nurse who picked up and held the butterfly for the widowed family member, there is no algorithm for doing such things. It is a matter of being open to intuition... creative spirit... energy field of intent... Spirit working through you... God... the Universe... Higher Power... or whatever it is that is comfortable in your own language and world view. It is the package of intention and presence that positions us to connect with this flow.

Energy endures

A final example of why intention and presence are important in spiritual care is that the energy that emanates from our meaningful connections with other people endures.

In Chapter 6, one of the reasons I suggested that the expression of positive qualities of character is important is because it "puts distinct energy out into the world, and this energy spreads and endures." You will recall the story of the Penn Center photograph of the former slave boy, capturing an enduring moment of grace during the Civil War.

Same idea here. Our intentional and present connections with other people puts energy out there that has a way of enduring long after the fact. An elderly woman recalls:

The year after my stroke was one of the hardest times in my life. I felt so out of control, initially hardly being able to move and speak and then having a long road back. I'm still not back where I was. I spent months doing painful rehab, mostly taking me away from my family and my normal life. I remember that I wondered for a long time if I would ever recover and there were some dark nights when I wasn't sure that it was all worth it.

What ultimately saved me was my ancestors. My grandparents were all kindly people who always told me I was special and always seemed to take such delight in seeing me. They'd look me right in the eye and were so interested in what I was doing, even if what a seven or eight-year-old girl was interested in couldn't have been real exciting to them.

They've all been gone for what... fifty years? But, you know... I could still feel them caring about me... loving me... and that love really kept me going during the dark times.

May we recognize and celebrate the enduring nature of the energy of caring and human connection that we put out there, as well.

CULTIVATING INTENTION AND PRESENCE

Let's consider some approaches to nurturing the qualities of healing intention and presence.

Be well

I am a long-time fan of *A Prairie Home Companion*. The spirit of the fictional characters who populate Lake Wobegon, Minnesota appeals to me... earnest, a little naïve and not always quite getting it, with a core of goodness. My interest in *PHC* has directed me to another Garrison Keillor media venture, *A Writer's Almanac*, on National Public Radio. When I am able to listen to this (which is not often, with the awkward schedule in my market area), I enjoy the comments on literary figures, the daily poem and the signature closing, "Be well, do good work, and keep in touch.®"

This is a pretty good formula. It links well-being with good work and with meaningful personal connections.

I believe that our personal orientation to intention and presence does indeed start with being well. Certainly, the alternative to being well is an impediment to intention and presence; when we are preoccupied, out of balance, overwhelmed, or bitter... it is difficult to manufacture genuine healing intention. Mark Twain's comment that "the most important thing is sincerity... if you can fake that, you've got it made" is a great one-liner, but rings hollow in the setting of real human suffering.

I recall a conversation with a psychiatrist colleague who asserted that "psychiatrists [and presumably other caring professionals] don't necessarily live any more effectively than anybody else... they just pull it together to use the skills that they have learned to work with other people." I disagree. I think that the privilege and honor of journeying with other people require us to be accountable for our own spiritual well-being beyond the point that would be required in other lines of work. I know from my experience in one of my past lives as a carpenter in New Hampshire that you can frame a building or roof a house without any particular spiritual grounding or focus, but it is not so in ministering to human suffering.

This is not to say that providing spiritual care requires us to be perfectly pure or angelic. With the possible exceptions of Mother Teresa, the Pope, and Red Sox designated hitter David Ortiz, all of us are fallible. We are not immune from struggles with mood and relationship difficulties and occasional thoughtless words, but I believe that we have a sacred trust to tend to our own wellness and centeredness in a devoted and persevering way.

What does this mean? This is a very large question. The field of psychology and behavioral health in the last century has seen hundreds... thousands... of frameworks for well-being, personal integration, self-actualization, fulfillment, identity formation and other such processes. Our spiritual and theological traditions touching on the journeys toward spiritual maturity and enlightenment extend back additional centuries and millennia.

Resilience

No one is immune or protected from challenges. We have too much work. We get sick. Other people don't treat us the way we might wish. The stock market goes up and down. Your candidate loses. Sometimes, serious abuses or accidents take place. We typically have very little control over "outside" challenges such as these.

We can, however, cultivate ways to live with balance, dignity, and even joy in spite of the outside challenges that come at us. Psychological research calls this "resilience," and identifies a number of approaches that have been found to help us to be resilient to life challenges, including:

Eating right. Amount (Americans eat twice as much as we should), type (colorful food, si, processed food, no) and reasons (food preparation and consumption is to enjoy).

Sleeping enough. Whatever is normal and restoring for you.

Exercising. Out of breath, 20 minutes, 3-5 times a week.

Making choices based on your values. Invest your time and your heart on what is important. Say no to what is not important. When you have to do something that is not important, do an acceptable job and move on.

Saying how you feel... but not dwelling on it. You have to talk about the hard things, but also be aware that what comes out of your mouth tends to become your reality.

Developing a spiritual practice. Prayer. Meditation. Journaling. Worship. Reading devotional material. Spending quiet time in some sacred place. Spiritual practices have a number of biological and emotional benefits and help you to stay focused on what really matters in your life.

Being charitable with yourself. Hold yourself to the same standards you would hold for someone else whom you dearly love.

Being open to wonder. Flowers and leaves coming out on the spring. Your body completely and automatically healing a cut. Sending a letter to Uncle Floyd in Hog Gulch, Tennessee for 42 cents and knowing that it will arrive. Watching a parent's loving touch of a young child. Watching a child's loving touch of an elderly parent.

Being grateful. Keep some account of the small and not so small blessings in your life.

Cultivating relationships. Be in touch, stay in touch, with people whom you love.

Being part of a community. Know and be known by other people whose journey coincides with yours.

Cultivating creativity and passions. Make some time to learn about something, or to create something that never existed before. Music. Writing. Poetry. Visual arts. Crafts. Hobbies. Cooking. Gardening. Bird watching. Salamander sleuthing. You get the idea.

Being where you are. Not yesterday. Not tomorrow. Not Hog Gulch. Not when Biff is finally potty trained. Not when you have been promoted to Regional Vice President. Where you are, now.

Trusting in the process. What if the Universe really brings people and circumstances into your life for a reason? What if you approached your life as if the Universe did this?

Rather than presuming to review this collective wisdom over the centuries, let me direct your attention to the table on resilience.

This is a one-page handout I put together three or four years ago that summarizes some of the psychological literature about resilience. As you will see, "resilience" in this context really has to do with wellness, balance, purpose and connections. I give this to people with the invitation to "review the list, see what resonates with you and plan some specific ways of following up on one or two areas." A few comments:

- **Mind-body-spirit.** Physical wellness goes hand in hand with emotional and spiritual wellness. In working with patients and professionals over the years, I have found very robust effects of pursuits that are grounded in the physical life, particularly exercise, nutrition, sleep and techniques of breathing. Indeed, my experience is that people who see me who get going on specific daily programs of walking or going to the gym, and who make some commitment to eat a little better, report better progress than people who do not tend to these areas. Hence, the reference at the top of this handout to nutrition, sleep and exercise.

  Speaking of mind-body-spirit approaches, by the way, I have also begun to recommend 4-7-8 breathing exercises to many people who see me. This is a simple and concrete technique that is centuries old and comes to me on the advice of some of my Arizona colleagues. Breathe in to a count of "4," hold it to a count of "7," and exhale to a count of "8." Three reps, three times daily. You can go to Google for more good information about the rationale and the technique.

- **Balance.** I think it is fair to say that a theme that flows through most approaches to well-being, and this particular take on resilience, involves balance. Everything in moderation. Balancing work and down time. Time with people and time alone. Time to be serious and time to be ridiculous.

Time to be active and time to be still. Time to realistically plan for the future, and time to be where you are right now.

- **Purpose and qualities of character.** (Ahem). A reminder that personal wellness and wholeness involves the nurturing of personal purpose and mission and of personally meaningful qualities of character, as we have considered in Chapters 5 and 6.

- **Gratitude.** I want to particularly emphasize the importance on the list of gratitude. The ability to go through the day with a spirit of gratefulness... being awake to goodness... is profoundly important. Albert Einstein is quoted: "There are two ways of living your life; one, as if nothing is a miracle, the other, as if everything is a miracle."

As an undergraduate at Dartmouth, there were certainly ample opportunities to study ponderous academic subjects with some nationally and world-renowned teachers. Analytic philosophy, Etruscan art, quantum mechanics, perspectives on the nation-state throughout history. Even amid this wealth of resources, the very best college course I took was a studio art course. The professor was the noted sculptor Varujan Bogosian, whose artistic niche is in the assemblage of familiar objects in novel contextual relationships. His gift to me and to the class was to help us to awaken to the beauty of the everyday objects and images that we all take for granted. Particularly memorable was a 20 minute, spontaneous, wondrous, reflection on the hinge. What a wonderful object is the hinge, he said... with its inherent unfolding shape and its ability to expand our relationship with space. This is gratitude; the ability to awaken to the present and emerging beauty of life.

The alternative to gratitude, by the way, is either dullness or cynicism. Dullness... the non-aware plodding through daily life... leaves us disconnected from Einstein's miracles. Cynicism infuses our own spirit and the world around us with toxic energy.

We will explore gratitude in greater detail in Chapter 10.

STRATEGY 7
Be well

As a context or foundation for cultivating intention and presence, consider the many dimensions of being-well that are important to you. You can

- Use the resilience handout as a template. Or you can use the CAMPS framework from Chapter 1 as a template.
- Use some other template that is familiar and comfortable for you.
- Reflect on how you think of wellness as you take this up with patients.
- Just think about your own life and pay attention to your wisdom and intuition.

What do you take pride in with regard to your own journey of wellness? What are you doing now that you can affirm?

What are the areas that you could stand to strengthen, to which you could devote more energy and attention? What differences would it make if you were to do this?

Among the ideas you have had about areas you could strengthen, what would be some next steps? To what would you commit yourself to further enhance your overall balance and mind-body-spirit well-being?

Be mindful

In Chapter 6, we considered "present awareness" of meaningful qualities of character. We explored some strategies... journaling, periodic check-in, retreats and community... for maintaining and enlivening this awareness.

The same challenge pertains for intention and presence; to maintain the current awareness of our intention as healers and our commitment to be present to people.

Some approaches to consider:

- **Devotional practices.**
  - Reading of sacred texts or other uplifting writing. Many spiritual traditions have daily resources for study and meditation.
  - Prayer or meditation.
  - Listening to spiritually centering music

- **Energy practices.** Tai Chi, yoga. I have always imagined that the experience of doing tai chi with 500 other people at 6AM in a municipal park in China must be energizing and inspirational. Lacking 500 other people or a municipal park in China, one can also pursue such energy practices privately. There are many good DVD programs and broadcast programs in early morning slots. As you develop some familiarity with such approaches, you can configure them to your own situation. I sometimes do a brief excerpt of a tai chi form before a half day of seeing patients, for instance.

- **Mini-meditation.** One of the Five Pillars of Islam is *Salah*, the daily ritual of prayer. Observant Muslims pray at five prescribed times; dawn, mid-day, late-afternoon, sunset and nightfall, reciting verses from the Qur'an, followed by optional personal prayers. Similarly, many religious traditions have the custom of grace (etymology; *gratia*, gratitude) as a blessing before meals.

These markers, set amid the daily rhythms of life, provide regular opportunities to become re-focused and spiritually centered.

In my professional life, I engage in daily markers or mini-meditations like this in two ways. As I have mentioned, I sometimes follow a beginning-of-the-day (or "beginning of the half day") practice of attenuated tai chi or brief reflection.

In addition to this, I have faithfully followed the Stairway Ritual for many years. The building where I work has two floors. It is built into a hillside, leading from higher ground down to the Kennebec River. Each of the floors has a level entrance, such that the distance between floors is determined by the pitch of the hillside. This is fairly substantial, such that there are 28 steps between the floors.

My office, where I see patients, is on the lower floor. The waiting room, where patients check in and from where I retrieve them for visits with me, is on the first floor. Being a tall, long-legged basketball player, my default approach to stairs is to bound up two at a time. The Stairway Ritual is that I deliberately take the last seven or eight steps up when I go to meet patients one at a time, using that brief period to clear my mind and soul of distractions and to remember... like the family physician at the beginning of this chapter... why I want to be present to the person I am about to see.

This makes a difference for me. It is a way of grounding myself in intention and healing presence that brings a little of The Sacred into my daily routine, and takes virtually no additional time.

Mini-meditations... I suspect that you may have some similar rituals with more dignified names... are particularly suited to daily transitions. For me, it is the beginnings of half days and the transitions to new patients. It may also be moving from clinical work to administrative work, or vice versa. Or moving from work to home or vice versa. Or beginning a session of writing part of a book.

STRATEGY 8
Pursue a practice of re-focusing and renewal during the day

Develop... renew... cultivate... a mindful practice of spiritual centering during the day, with particular attention to intention and presence. Experiment with devotional practices, energy practices, or mini-meditations.

Consider: how do you best make this a part of the rhythm of your daily routine? How might such practices fit into the transitions that you experience? How do you best re-focus your intention and presence? How much do you experience these practices as re-connecting with your own commitments, and/or as being open to wisdom and energy from the larger spiritual world within you or beyond you?

Hold on to affirmations

I have always had great admiration and respect for 12-step programs. Alcoholics Anonymous and spin-offs (Alanon, Narcotics Anonymous, Overeaters Anonymous, Gamblers Anonymous, among others) offer a rich source of community and wisdom for people changing their lives.

A distinctive vehicle for the wisdom of 12-step programs has been a large collection of aphorisms, or pithy reminders about key ideas for recovery. You see some of the more prominent aphorisms on iridescent bumper stickers and hear a lot more by listening to people who live them. Examples include:

- Easy does it
- Let go and let God
- One day at a time
- First things first
- You have to give it away in order to keep it

Distilling personally-meaningful wisdom into short and memorable aphorisms is another helpful approach to maintaining present awareness of purpose, mission, qualities of character, and the energy of intention and presence.

For a number of years, my faculty role at the University of Arizona School of Medicine has involved teaching a Web-based module on spirituality as part of the two-year fellowship in integrative medicine at the Arizona Center for Integrative Medicine.[17] One of my two colleagues in teaching this module is Dr. Howard

Silverman, a family physician and long-time medical educator. Howard's content contribution to this module is in the areas of ceremony, ritual and affirmations. His idea of affirmations is very much along the lines of 12-step aphorisms... succinct distillation of wisdom and intention that help to focus our daily journeys. He comments, "Personal affirmations are a simple way to elevate the integrative physician's awareness of self, patient and circumstances. By acting as a reminder to focus one's attention on one's intention, they act almost as a post-hypnotic suggestion. Practical experience is that over a period of time, one's wishes really can come true!"

The particular exercise that Dr. Silverman suggests to our integrative medicine fellows is to a) identify a specific group of patients or visit types that are especially difficult, and b) design a personal affirmation to help with these patients. Some examples are in the table on the following pages.

I have seen hundreds of these affirmations over the last few years and I never fail to be impressed. They are rich, creative, and very personal.

STRATEGY 9
Create a personal affirmation

Develop your own personal affirmation in the format that Dr. Silverman recommends. Describe a category of patients or patient encounters or, for that matter, other situations that you find challenging in your professional life. Create an affirmation that succinctly captures what you would like to hold in your mind and your heart as you face these challenges. Review this daily.

Affirmations
from the Fellowship in Integrative Medicine,
Arizona Center for Integrative Medicine

A specific group of patients or visit types that are especially difficult:

Patients that are in pain but are also looking for more medication and sometimes manipulate me to get what they want

A personal affirmation to help with these patients:

I will have a touchstone in my pocket that I rub before going into a difficult patient's room, reminding me to have compassion and understanding but to not allow my own well being to disappear and let others take advantage of me.

A specific group of patients or visit types that are especially difficult:

Patients that have so many issues and are by nature tangential in their communication. I often find myself losing my ability to listen to them and move into the "do" mode.

A personal affirmation to help with these patients:

I will stay grounded with all patients in order for me to learn the true reason for their visit. I will stay grounded so that their need will be revealed to me.

A specific group of patients or visit types that are especially difficult:

Chronic pain patients that demand narcotics and in general, patients who expect you as the physician to heal them without expecting that they will need to put in any of the work.

A personal affirmation to help with these patients:

I will view these patients as having missed the opportunity of development in their lives that empowers them to self-heal; they lack the innate wisdom that often comes through introspection. Be patient and understanding, guide toward inner wisdom.

A specific group of patients or visit types that are especially difficult:

Overweight patients, and all the resulting medical problems, present particular challenges for me. I get frustrated when I think they are not motivated to change and seem to take a passive and resistant approach to their life.

A personal affirmation to help with these patients:

If I become frustrated with a patient, I honor my own frustration and recognize that it comes out of my desire to see this person change. I recognize that I want them to do what I want, not appreciating that the struggles that challenge them also give them their unique character. When I recognize my desire to change them, I sit back, breathe, and engage in deep listening. Rather that trying to get them to see my point of view and lecturing them, I engage with them in the fullness of life and find out more about what makes them who they are. My frustration lessens because I alter my focus and intention. Instead of trying to get them to change, I am listening to them and their concerns.

A specific group of patients or visit types that are especially difficult:

Angry, sullen, obstreperous, drunk, etc... patients. Hmm... that's a lot of our ER patients!

A personal affirmation to help with these patients:

Anybody can be a teacher. The most difficult people can be the best teachers. The most difficult moments can be the best opportunities to learn.

SUMMARY

- Personal spiritual well-being (groundedness, wholeness, centeredness, aliveness) supports personal equanimity and helps us to provide creative, quality spiritual care.
- Grounding ourselves in healing intention and presence is a key approach that promotes personal spiritual well-being.
- We ground ourselves in healing intention and presence by
  - cultivating personal health and resilience
  - creating rituals and practices that promote mindfulness
  - developing and holding personal affirmations.

REFERENCES

1. Shealey N, Church D. *Soul Medicine: Awakening Your Inner Blueprint for Abundant Health and Energy.* Santa Rosa, CA: Elite; 2006.
2. Nash C. Psychokinetic control of bacterial growth. *Am J Psychical Res.* 1982;51:217-221.
3. Nash C. Test of psychokinetic control of bacterial mutation. *J Am Soc Psychical Res.* 1984;78(2):145-152.
4. Bengston W, Krinsley D. The effect of the "laying on of hands" on transplanted breast cancer in mice. *J Sci Exploration.* 2000;14(3):353-364.
5. Mehl-Madrona L. Connectivity and healing: Some hypotheses about the phenomenon and how to study it. *Advances Mind Body Med.* 2005;21(1):12-28.
6. Harris W, Gowda M, Kolb J, et al. A randomized, controlled trial of the effects of remote, intercessory prayer on outcomes in patients admitted to the coronary care unit. *Arch Intern Med.* 1999;159(19):2273-2278.
7. Bryd R. Positive therapeutic effects of intercessory prayer in a coronary care unit population. *Southern Med J.* 1988;81:826-829.
8. Sicher F, Targ E, Moore D, Smith H. A randomized double-blind study of the effect of distant healing in a population with advanced AIDS - report of a small-scale study. *West J Med.* 1998;169(6).
9. Astin J, Harkness E, Ernst E. The efficacy of "distant healing:" A systematic review of randomized trials. *Ann Int Med.*

2000;132(11):903-910.

10. Crawford C, Sparber A, Jonas W. A systematic review of the quality of research on hands-on and distant healing: Clinical and laboratory studies. *Alt Ther.* 2003;9(3):A96-A104.

11. Hubble M, Duncan B, Miller S. *The Heart & Soul of Change: What Works in Therapy.* Washington, DC: American Psychological Association; 1999.

12. Friedman E. *Generation to Generation: Family Process in Church and Synagogue.* New York: Guilford; 1985.

13. Churchill L, Schenck D. Healing skills for medical practice. *Ann Int Med.* 2008;149(10):720-724.

14. Laidlaw T, Kaufman D, Sargeant J, MacLeod H, Blake K, Simpson D. What makes a physician an exemplary communicator with patients? *Patient Educ Couns.* 2007;68(2):153-160.

15. McDonough-Means S, Kreitzer M, Bell I. Fostering a healing presence and investigating its mediators. *J Alt Comp Med.* 2004;10(Supplement 1):S25-S41.

16. Dyer W. *The Power of Intention.* Carlsbad, CA: Hay House; 2004.

17. Craigie FC, Jr., Silverman H, Maizes V. Teaching spirituality on the Web: Experiences from the University of Arizona Associate Fellowship in Integrative Medicine. *Explore!* 2007;16(2):56-62.

CLINICAL:
CONNECTIONS WITH WHAT
MATTERS TO YOUR PATIENTS

In the previous three chapters, we have explored the personal arena of spiritual care. Our own centeredness, intention, and presence are in themselves good spiritual care, and also lay the foundation for more specific clinical approaches. The following three chapters explore these more specific clinical approaches.

You will recall our definition of spiritual care from Chapter 3: "helping people to connect with the things that really matter to them." This is the task of spiritual care in the clinical arena; to understand what really matters to our patients (what is "vital and sacred," in Koop's phrase) and to support them in giving it life.

We will consider a variety of approaches to spiritual inquiry in Chapter 8. In Chapter 9, we will explore some ways of organizing conversations with people to identify solutions... bringing together patients' wisdom and our wisdom... to help them in their journeys. In Chapter 10, we will look specifically at transcendence and valued directions.

Chapter Eight

Pick One or Two Areas to Inquire about People's Spirituality

At the heart of being a ministering person
is seeking to hear and understand
the story of the suffering person standing before us
and to encourage hope in that person
in developing the next chapter of the story[1]

Verna Benner Carson and Harold Koenig, MD

In Chapter 2, I proposed four reasons why spirituality is important in health and wellness care. Spirituality is intimately related to health, wholeness and well-being. Spirituality mediates choices in health behaviors. Spirituality often frames the ways that people cope with adversity and pursue the journey toward wellness/wholeness. And spirituality is important because people want to be known in this way by their caregivers.

Consider some patients that many of us work with:

- a 60 year old man with chronic Hepatitis C and cirrhosis who is approaching the end of his life
- a 23 year old woman who is pregnant for the first time

- a 45 year old woman with a recurrence of ovarian cancer
- a 79 year old man who has had a stroke that leaves him with a substantial expressive deficit
- an 18 year old young man who needs a college physical
- a 39 year old woman who smokes and has borderline hypertension
- a 28 year old man with chronic back pain and oxycodone dependence

Wholistic practitioner that you are, you recognize that spirituality may be important to these people for the several reasons we have considered. What, specifically, would you wish to know about their spirituality and how will you pursue this? Do you raise the subject of spirituality or do you allow them to do so? What words do you use?

In this chapter, we will consider some specific approaches to spiritual inquiry. I prefer the term, "inquiry," to the term, "assessment," by the way. "Assessment," to me, connotes a detached and impersonal process, not unlike assessing why the oxygen sensor in your car's exhaust system continues to blow out. "Inquiry," on the other hand, connotes a more engaged, relational process.

Our modern word "inquiry," like "inquire" and "query," comes from the Latin word "quaerere," meaning "to seek." "Seeking," I think, has a much richer presence than "asking" or "assessing." Spiritual inquiry really grows out of a spirit of inquisitiveness… or curiosity… or seeking… about what it is like to be somebody else. You may choose any variety of specific questions to explore people's spirituality, but ultimately it is this spirit of inquiry and seeking, of honoring people by the commitment to really understand what matters to them, that makes it work.

And an additional word of preface; spiritual inquiry, with spiritual "intervention," is a fluid process. It is not cleanly compartmentalized and sequential. We will consider *mostly* spiritual inquiry in this chapter and *mostly* spiritual conversations directed toward change in the next chapter, but this is not to say that these projects are separate and sequential. They are not.

When I was doing my training as a psychologist in the Late Bronze Age, my colleagues and I were taught that there was "assessment" and then there was "intervention." First, you did an assessment, then you formulated a plan and conducted the intervention. You asked clients a long list of questions about presenting complaint, symptoms, psychiatric history, social history, family history and other items, then formulated a 5-axis DSM diagnosis, then mapped out a treatment plan.

This compartmentalized and sequential model may fit for some of the settings in which we work with people. A specialty consultation in Integrative Medicine, for instance, may often begin with a comprehensive exploration of people's lives, leading to the development of a menu of options for integrative care (mind-body approaches, nutritional approaches, botanicals, energy work, and so forth).

In many of the settings of health and wellness care where we see people, however, the conversation is much more fluid and directed toward change as opportunities arise.

Clinician: When you were talking about caring for your crotchety grandfather in the last year of his life, I thought I was hearing a lot of patience and kindness.

Patient: Yeah, I think I did pretty well by him.

Clinician: I have used the words "patience" and "kindness." How would you put into words the kind of person that you tried to be with your grandfather?

Patient: I was patient... that's right... I don't know, I guess I try not to get too hung up on people's behavior and I try to find some goodness underneath somewhere.

Clinician: Wow, "goodness underneath somewhere." How do you see yourself doing with the "goodness underneath somewhere" in your life right now?

This example is spiritual inquiry, *and* it is spiritual intervention. It is *inquiry* insofar as the clinician is looking for personal values or qualities of character that the patient expresses during some good times. It is *intervention* in two ways; it is affirming and it is inviting. First, the clinician is focusing this part of the conversation on the patient's positive spiritual values, thereby affirming this part of the patient's life experience. Second, the clinician is inviting the patient to think about how she is doing with these values right now, thereby inviting her into the present awareness, connection, and expression of these values in her current life.

TWO TYPES OF SPIRITUAL INQUIRY

The world of spiritual inquiry (unlike Gaul) is divided into two parts; inventories and conversation. You write it down or you talk about it. I want to review both of these approaches, with particular reference to a perspective on conversational spiritual inquiry that I have developed over a number of years.

Spirituality inventories

Behavioral scientists love inventories. There are thousands of inventories measuring every conceivable human state, trait and experience.

In the realm of spirituality, there are a goodly number of inventories that measure beliefs, experiences and practices having to do with spirituality and religion. Most ask respondents to rate the importance or frequency of particular items on Likert scales ("I feel an awareness of God's presence... never, rarely, occasionally, frequently, always"). Some, particularly the older inventories, are theistic, while others are more inclusive. Most paper and pencil inventories have been developed and utilized in research settings, although some may aspire to have clinical applications.

In the sidebar on the next page, I highlight a few spirituality inventories that are relatively prominent in the literature of spirituality and health and health care. Historically, the forerunner in this field is the Spiritual Well-Being Scale. I'm not sure anyone is counting, but it is safe to say that this inventory has appeared

Self-report inventories of spirituality

Inventory

FACIT-Sp-12[1]
Year: 2002
# of items: 12
Theistic: No
Aggregate score: Yes
Illustrative item: *My illness has strengthened my faith or spiritual beliefs*
Comments: Oncology: from Functional Assessment of Cancer Therapy projects
                         Two of 12 items relate to reactions to illness.

Spirituality Index of Well-Being[2]
Year: 2004
# of items: 12
Theistic: No
Aggregate score: Yes
Illustrative item: *I haven't yet found my life's purpose.*
Comments: Self-efficacy subscale and life scheme subscale
                         Negatively worded items (I don't know... There is not much I can do)

Spiritual Involvement and Beliefs Scale[3]
Year: 1998
# of items: 26
Theistic: No (A power greater than myself)
Aggregate score: Yes
Illustrative item: *My spiritual life fulfills me in ways that material possessions do not.*
Comments: Purposefully "generic" wording
                         Developed as tools for clinicians (like mental status) and research

Beliefs and Values Scale[4]
Year: 2006
# of items: 20
Theistic: Yes (God)
Aggregate score: Yes
Illustrative item: *I believe God is an all pervading presence.*
Comments: Standardized on broad range of patients and non-patients.

INSPIRIT: Index of Core Spiritual Experiences[5]
Year: 1991
# of items: 7 (last of which asks whether people have had 12 spiritual experiences)
Theistic: Yes (God)
Aggregate score: Yes
Illustrative item: *Do you agree or disagree: "God dwells within you."*
Comments: Developed by chaplain, seminarian and medical student
                         Six questions about attitudes and practices in addition to the last item

Spiritual Perspective Scale[6]
Year: 1987
# of items: 10
Theistic: Yes (God or a higher power)
Aggregate score: Yes
Illustrative item: *Spirituality is a significant part of my life.*
Comments: Behavior and beliefs subscales
                         Goal to advance understanding of spirituality/health relationships

1. Peterman AH, Fitchett G, Brady MJ, Hernandez L, Cella D. Measuring spiritual well-being in people with cancer: The Functional Assessment of Chronic Illness Therapy- Spiritual Well-Being Scale (FACIT-Sp). *Annals of Beh Med.* 2002;24(1):49-58.
2. Daaleman T, Frey B. The spirituality index of well-being: A new instrument for health-related quality-of-life research. *Arch Fam Med.* 2004;2:499-503.
3. Hatch RL, Burg MA, Naberhaus DS, Hellmich LK. The Spiritual Involvement and Beliefs Scale. Development and testing of a new instrument. *J Fam Pract.* Jun 1998;46(6):476-486.
4. King M, Jones L, Barnes K, et al. Measuring spiritual belief: development and standardization of a Beliefs and Values Scale. *Psychol Med.* 2006;36(3):417-425.
5. VandeCreek L, Ayres S, Bassham M. Using INSPIRIT to conduct spiritual assessments. *J Pastoral Care.* Spring 1995;49(1):83-89.
6. Dailey D, Stewart A. Psychometric characteristics of the spiritual perspective scale in pregnant African-American women. *Res Nurs Health.* 2007;30(1):61-71.

in research since its development in 1983 more frequently than any other instrument, and it often shows up as a validity standard for newer instruments. The authors... as is certainly their prerogative... also keep it tightly wrapped; as far as I am aware, the instrument is not available for viewing in the published literature or on the Web. Copies may be purchased (from $2.25 to $1.00, depending on quantity) from their website.

Among the several well-conceived inventories in the sidebar, two recent instruments particularly appeal to me; the FACIT-Sp[2] and the Spiritual Perspective Scale.[3] The former was developed and is used in oncology settings; the latter has been used in exploring the spirituality of various demographic cohorts, such as pregnant African-American women in the study that I cite. Both of these inventories are short, suitable for people with low to modest literacy and above, touch on important spiritual issues (meaning, closeness to God or higher power, purpose in life, strengthening of faith or spiritual beliefs from illness, etc.) and are developed with thorough attention to methodological and statistical standards.

I consider spirituality inventories to be primarily useful for research. As Dailey and Stewart say of the Spiritual Perspective Scale, "Accurate measurement of spirituality can advance understanding of its link to health, which can lead to the development and testing of nursing interventions to improve health and well-being."[3] (p. 69) These instruments give us a clearer view of spirituality/health relationships with groups of people and can assist in evaluating how spiritual interventions in nursing and other fields affect people's spiritual well-being.

The clinical applications of these instruments are limited. Generally, I think that they are too cumbersome for routine use in clinical settings... for which most of them were not designed, anyway. It is easy to be overloaded with data, with the clinical and, probably, ethical imperative to respond to responses that you get. You will have patients' responses to a dozen or more intriguing statements or questions. "I feel that God has abandoned me... (often)." "There is a clear purpose for my life... (usually)." "My faith brings me comfort in the face of illness… (sometimes)." Given that you have asked patients to reveal their perspectives on personal items such as these, they all merit further conversation… which may or may not be possible.

I also believe, as I have described, that personal issues are better addressed in person.

There are, however, two ways of using inventories such as these that can be clinically viable. First, these inventories can be completed by patients and subsequently reviewed with clinicians. VandeCreek and colleagues, for instance, suggest that students of pastoral care could leave the INSPIRIT with patients on first pastoral visits and then discuss the results on subsequent visits.[4] I think that this approach is best suited to spiritual care specialists (like students of pastoral care) or to specialized health care settings like Hospice.

Second, these inventories can be offered to patients as resources for personal reflection. As an example, the INSPIRIT inventory was also reprinted with self-scoring instructions in the popular magazine *Spirituality and Health* in the context of inviting readers to reflect on how their spirituality supports personal resilience.[5]

Conversational templates

The other approach to spiritual inquiry is conversation.

There have been three principle templates… acronyms…for organizing conversational spiritual inquiry. The earliest among them is the SPIRITual History, from family physician Todd Maugans, then at the University of Virginia.[6] The acronym stands for:

- **S**piritual belief systems (religious affiliation or belief systems)
- **P**ersonal spirituality (importance and particulars of personal beliefs and practices)
- **I**ntegration with a spiritual community (involvement and roles in spiritual or religious groups)
- **R**itualized practices and restrictions (spiritual practices associated with spiritual community or belief systems)

- **I**mplications for medical care (how patients hope that spiritual life might be incorporated in health care)
- **T**erminal events planning (influence of spirituality in end of life care)

Dr. Maugans suggested a number of possible situations for conversation using this template, including serious illnesses, perioperative periods, and health maintenance examinations. He also proposed that history-taking with this template could be done in single settings in the case of more intense clinical issues, or over a period of time, with responses collected in a special section of the medical record.

A second template was developed a few years later under the leadership of family physician Gowri Anandarajah at Brown.[7] The HOPE acronym stands for:

- Sources of **H**ope, meaning, comfort, strength, peace, love and connection
- **O**rganized religion (participation in religious or spiritual community)
- **P**ersonal spirituality and **P**ractices (meaningful personal spiritual beliefs and practices)
- **E**ffects on medical care and end-of-life issues (effects of illness on spirituality and implications for medical care)

As with the Maugans framework, Dr. Anandarajah suggests specific conversational approaches to pursue these several areas.

The most widely disseminated template for conversational spiritual inquiry comes from Christina Puchalski, who is Director of the George Washington Institute for Spirituality and Health at George Washington University. A physician practicing internal medicine and geriatrics, Dr. Puchalski has been an international leader in advocacy and development of educational resources about spirituality for medical professionals. Her FICA template is presented in the sidebar.[8] This has appeared in numerous publications and has been a centerpiece of spirituality curricula in medical education programs at the undergraduate and postgraduate level.

You will see common themes among the three templates, particularly with respect to personal spiritual beliefs and practices, engagement with spiritual communities, and the implications of patients' spirituality for their health care. In each case, the premise

---

FICA

Christina Puchalski, MD
George Washington Institute for Spirituality and Health

F – Faith and Belief

Do you consider yourself spiritual or religious?" or "Do you have spiritual beliefs that help you cope with stress?" If the patient responds "No," the health care provider might ask, "What gives your life meaning?" Sometimes patients respond with answers such as family, career, or nature.

I – Importance

"What importance does your faith or belief have in our life? Have your beliefs influenced how you take care of yourself in this illness? What role do your beliefs play in regaining your health?"

C – Community

"Are you part of a spiritual or religious community? Is this of support to you and how? Is there a group of people you really love or who are important to you?" Communities such as churches, temples, and mosques, or a group of like-minded friends can serve as strong support systems for some patients.

A – Address in Care

"How would you like me, your healthcare provider, to address these issues in your healthcare?"

---

is that the clinician will be guided by the content areas signified by the pieces of the acronyms, but will also have the flexibility to follow directions in interviews that would be clinically important.

I think that these templates can potentially be very helpful for clinicians in health and wellness care. As I suggested in the Introduction, I believe that one of the main impediments to embracing and exploring spirituality in health care is fear… that we will become lost, overwhelmed, or will not know how to proceed. Structure helps. Having a map or template can reduce the discomfort associated with uncertainty.

The particular content areas of these templates, moreover, seem to me to be very much on target. What is somebody's view of the world and their personal spiritual orientation? How does this help them? In what ways have they been meaningfully connected with compatriots who share some of their spiritual journey? How does their spirituality influence their approach to health care? How would they hope that their spirituality would be a part of their health care?

STRATEGY 10

Use conversational templates for spiritual inquiry

Choose one (or more) among the SPIRITual History, HOPE and FICA. Interview your partner, or some friends or colleagues, and some patients. Get a sense of how the conversation flows and what are the components that are most germane for your setting.

PRACTICAL CLINICAL APPROACHES TO SPIRITUAL INQUIRY

I want to consider now some practical clinical approaches that I find useful with issues such as these; the "what," "when" and "how" of spiritual inquiry. First, let me emphasize a point about templates and paradigms.

What is important is to find or develop some template... some structure for thinking about and guiding conversations about spirituality... that works for you. I am less interested in your pursuing any of the particular templates that we have considered, or my own CAMPS framework that I am about to revisit with you, than I am in your developing ways of framing these questions that fit with your own style, language, temperament and cultural setting.

In the arena of evaluation of possible problems with alcohol, for instance, most of us have encountered Ewing's CAGE questionnaire... questions focusing on Cutting down, Annoyance by criticism, Guilty feelings, and Eye-openers.[9] This is a very helpful framework that I'm sure has informed the ways that many clinicians approach substance abuse issues. I find that most established clinicians, however, use this more in part than in whole, and often merge some of the CAGE questions with their own. I think that finding an approach to inquiry about possible alcohol issues that fits for individual clinicians is more important than whether or not clinicians use the particular CAGE framework. The key issue is being able to ask your own questions about alcohol with genuineness and confidence, and to have some sense of where you go with the answers you might receive.

Same thing with spirituality inquiry. I suspect that you *already* have some good approaches that you pursue to explore what matters to patients. Great. I want to affirm the experience and wisdom that you bring to this conversation, along with describing some approaches that help to guide the process of spiritual inquiry for me.

CAMPS

You will recall the introduction to CAMPS in Chapter 1… the framework of dimensions of spirituality named in honor of the uninsulated, rattle-trap structures in the Great North Woods of Maine where you go to restore your soul.

The sidebar on the next page presents a summary of what each of these five dimensions involves and presents some questions that may be used to explore them.

Picking and choosing questions. In the module on spirituality that I chair for the fellowship programs at the Arizona Center for Integrative Medicine, my colleague David Rychener, PhD invites the Fellows to interview someone using one of the templates that he presents… FICA, HOPE, the SPIRITual history, and CAMPS, among others. Many fellows chose to ask most of the questions from the CAMPS sidebar and the feedback we receive is that this is generally a helpful exercise.

CAMPS: A Framework for Conversations about Spirituality

C ommunity

Participation in a supportive community of people

Who are the people who are close to you?
What groups or organizations are you involved with?

A ctivities

Spiritually related activities that provide coherence and comfort
Ceremonies, sacraments, rituals
Prayer and devotional practices

What do you do to help yourself be more peaceful?
What do you do to help yourself be more centered?
What are the rituals or traditions that are meaningful for you?

M eaning and purpose

Using personal gifts, talents, skills or character on behalf of something that matters
Experience of significance, making a contribution to some larger good
Perception that one's life has value and worth
Suffering ... and hope

What are the things that are really important to you?
What do you take pride in?
What do you hope for?
Where do you find strength? What helps you to keep going?
What do you hope the legacy of your life will be?
What do you care about?

P assions

Being excited, passionate and engaged with some aspects of life
Experiencing joy

What do you find yourself getting really excited about?
What do you get really passionate about?
When do you find yourself engaged in something and lose track of time?

S pirit

Relationship with God, Spirit, Higher Power etc.

How is your relationship with God* important to your life and health?

* use language that patient uses (God, Higher Power) first

In practice, I never ask all of these questions in one sitting. I suppose one can do this... perhaps in a specialized setting such as Hospice... but my own approach is to pick and choose.

There are some among the CAMPS/sidebar questions that I ask most of the time when I get to know people. Probably the single area that I touch on with most people has to do with the arena of character strengths and virtues, as we reviewed in Chapter 6.

Fred (having asked about topics like nutrition, exercise and relaxing practices): *One of the things that I am always interested in with people is understanding what they take pride in, in terms of the kind of person that they try to be. How would you put into words some of what you have been proud about in living your life day to day?*
Patient: *Hm... I guess I try to help people.*
Fred: *Cool.* (Wanting to bring some of the energy of this quality into the conversation)... *What would be an example of how you have done this?*
Patient: *I have a next-door neighbor in her eighties...*

or

Fred: *One of the things that I am always interested in with people is understanding what they take pride in, in terms of the kind of person that they try to be. How would you put into words some of what you have been proud about in living your life day to day?*
Patient: *I dunno.*
Fred: *OK.* (Going from the example to the theme, rather than from the theme to the example)... *When has there been a time when you felt pretty good about yourself from something you had been doing?*
Patient: *Hm... I have this next-door neighbor in her eighties... she's sweet but she's unsteady a lot. I'll sweep her steps when it snows... sometimes I'll bring her milk or orange juice. Sometimes when I don't have a lot going on (which isn't very often), I'll just go over and hang out for a little while because I think she gets really lonely.*
Fred: *Cool. I can see from the way that you are describing it that*

looking out for her is something you take pride in…
Patient: *It's no big deal, anybody would do it.*
Fred: *OK… but I'm wondering as you talk about looking out for her, what that says about the kind of person that you try to be…*
Patient: *I guess I try to be helpful to people.*

When I ask about character strengths and virtues in this manner, by the way, the overwhelmingly most consistent response that I get is some variation of "helping people." Language from the last few weeks, for instance, has included "making people's lives better," "making a difference with people," and "contributing to society."

I suspect that if you were to look at transcripts of my interviews with people, there would be some variation over time in the particular CAMPS questions that I would introduce in conversations with patients. I will frequently also ask… in the "Community" domain, for instance… about kindred spirits. *"You're talking about how important your own 'spirituality' is to you… are you involved with a particular community of people who share these interests with you?"*

Picking up on patient experiences. As often as I *introduce* CAMPS questions into conversations, my asking CAMPS questions is prompted by what patients are saying… by the flow of their telling their stories. The CAMPS questions are an expression of curiosity and sometimes of wonder in picking up on their experiences.

I am continually fascinated and touched, for instance, by how people cope with hardship. There is no dearth of suffering among people that I see, and it is often a good gateway to understanding spirituality to explore what keeps people going.

I recently saw a 39 year old man, a single parent, whose stated problem was "anxiety and panic." As I inquired about some of his story, a tragic picture emerged. His former girlfriend, the mother of his two younger children, had been brutally murdered. Despondent, he had lapsed into drug use and the children were taken away by the girlfriend's mother and removed out of state. In spite of an eventual settlement that theoretically gave him joint custody and visitation privileges, the girlfriend's mother had withheld the children from him and blocked any attempts at his contacting them. He had, in the last couple of years, cleaned up his substance abuse, held down a job and been a solid dad to his high school son (by a previous relationship), but he said that not a day went by that he did not despair of the loss of these children. Some of the conversation:

Fred: *Wow, what an incredibly hard thing for a parent… what has kept you going through this?*
Patient: *My son.*
Fred: *Your son…*
Patient: *My son is the center of my life… I have to be there for him… I want to show him that I can still make somebody of myself even with all that's come down.*
Fred: *When you say "make somebody of myself," tell me more… help me to understand what that means to you…*
Patient: *Well, just not giving up is part of it… being a man my son can look up to… maybe I can show him something about what it means to be a man and to be a dad. I really want to better myself, too… go back to school, get a better job than the on and off stuff I've done.*

All of us would reflexively feel and express sympathy to this man as we hear his story. The additional step of exploring what keeps him going has quickly opened up a number of qualities and connections in his life that matter to him… that are "vital and sacred" for him. His love for his son, his wanting to make someone of himself, his wanting to better himself. All of these values will enrich his life, and probably substantially heal his struggle with anxiety, as he continues to pursue them.

I find that it is frequently very fruitful to take these extra steps when people report any kind of life change, perseverance, or "success" in what matters to them. I sometimes joke with our family medicine residents about the *"wow and how"* routine. The *"wow"* reflects the expression of affirmation and wonder for the efforts people have made in their lives, like the single parent in the story above. The *"how"* reflects the inquiry about what it was that enabled people to accomplish what they did. The "wow and how" routine pertains to patients who have:

- survived abuse (even if not perfectly)
- stopped drinking for 3 years between 1997 and 2000
- come to some reconciliation with a demeaning parent
- lost 9 pounds
- gone on with life in spite of having made some bad mistakes
- reduced their A1c level to 6.4
- become less depressed

Picking up on patient experiences and following up with CAMPS questions often can provide a good window on people's spirituality.

Language. *What is going on here? The word "spirituality" does not appear in the above transcript, yet you are holding this out as an example of spiritual care. What gives?*

Good questions. We talked in Chapter 1 about the idea that spirituality... what is "vital and sacred" in people's lives... may or may not be framed in spiritual or religious language.

In clinical conversations, similarly, what is vital and sacred, meaningful, and life-giving for people may or may not be framed in spiritual language.

My practice, in fact, is that I am very slow to introduce spirituality language in conversations with patients. First, I want interactions with patients to have a spirit or tone that is more "conversational" than "clinical." I am hesitant to introduce words that are not part of the common parlance of our interactions with one another. Ideally, the language we use with patients has to pass the "next door neighbor" test; if you wouldn't say it that way to your next door neighbor (assuming you didn't live next door to the recently-deceased William F. Buckley), don't say it. "What keeps you going," for instance, is phrasing I prefer to "What sustains you," or even "Where do you find meaning and purpose?" Plain English (or plain whatever-language-you-conduct-business-in) has a flow and disarming presence that clinical language does not.

The second reason why I am slow to introduce spirituality language is that I want the conversation to be anchored in language that is meaningful for patients, more than it is meaningful for me. I want patients to hold ownership of spiritual language.

In fact, with occasional exceptions, I am almost never the first person to introduce spirituality language in the conversation.

Fred: *This aching emptiness from the death of your son... what is your sense of how healing is going to happen for you?*
Patient: *Somehow I need to make peace with what happened... I need to let go.*
Fred: *Make peace... let go...* [gee whiz, I sound like Carl Rogers in Psych 101... it isn't usually like that, honest...]
Patient: *I need to make peace with the Universe.*
Fred: *OK, when you say "the Universe," tell me more what you mean... help me to understand...*

In this example, the phrase "the Universe" has personal meaning for this patient. My ongoing conversation with her, I believe, will be more fruitful (and more honorable) when it is grounded in her language, rather than in more generic spirituality language that comes from me.

The CAMPS question I give as an example in the previous section, by the way, ("What keeps you going?") is often a rich source of personally-meaningful spiritual language for patients. "My faith," "my spirituality," "the 12 steps," the Man Upstairs," and so forth.

This is a practice that I think is generally helpful in healing conversations. I had a patient some time ago whose presenting concern... what it said on the referral form... was "depression." Asking her how she would put into words what she would wish to be like instead of the way she had been, she said "smoother." As far as I know, there is no empirically-derived treatment recommendation for "smoothness," but I would rather anchor the conversation in this idiosyncratically-meaningful construct than I would in language and constructs that come from me. The conversation proceeds... what helps her to be smooth? When has she been smoother than other times and what do we learn from this? And when I see her back, the opening question is not "How depressed have you been?" It is "How smooth have you been?"

STRATEGY 11
Identify conversation-openers

Using resources of CAMPS questions, the conversational templates we have reviewed and your own wisdom and experience, identify one or two questions that you can use to open conversations about patients' spirituality. I have mentioned that questions like "What keeps you going," and "How were you successful in doing that," and "What is there about how you live your life that you are particularly proud about?" fit for my style and clinical/cultural setting. Identify some similar questions that fit with your own style and language, and with the setting in which you work.

WHEN IN THE COURSE OF HUMAN EVENTS

We have so far considered some practical approaches to *how* you conduct spiritual inquiry in clinical settings. Pick a template... or create your own template, or questions that fit for you and your setting. Introduce questions or pick up on leads that you hear from patients. Anchor the conversation in words and language that have personal meaning for patients.

Let's now consider the question of *when* to conduct some spiritual inquiry.

Well person visits

Visits without specific health complaints… meet-the-clinician visits, annual exams, paps, consultations about health maintenance or wellness… can be good times to insert some spiritual inquiry questions. My suggestion to our residents is to ask something that opens up the conversation about what matters to people.'

- *What do you take pride in?*
- *How would you put into words the kind of person that you try to be?*
- *When you are at your best, what does that look like?*
- *Where do you find joy?*
- *What helps you to be more peaceful and centered?*
- *What keeps you going in harder times?*
- *What do you turn to when you get down?*

The possibilities are limitless. I'm not sure that the particular question is as important as just the fact of raising the subject of what matters in somebody's life. Raising this subject in well person visits gives you information about what motivates and sustains people, and communicates to patients that this is a legitimate area that has a bearing on their health.

I think that this is particularly important in pediatric visits. For reasons of culture and social convention, it is so easy for parents to hold and express negative appraisals of their children. "He's ADD." "She never listens or minds." "He's more interested in stupid video games than reading." "She's in the Terrible Twos."

Asking specifically about positive qualities of character can reinforce parents' perceptions of strengths that they already see, and can sometimes help parents to see their children in new ways. "What is he especially good at?" "When has there been a time when you have been really proud of her?" "How would you put into words the best thing about the kind of person you see him becoming?"

Lifestyle change

As people wrestle with changes in health habits or practices, some spiritual inquiry can help to strengthen the foundation for their efforts.

You will recall the discussion of health goals and life goals in Chapter 2... that clarity about life goals (how you wish to be able to function and live your life) provides energy for health goals like changes in nutrition, exercise, smoking or substance abuse.

Bob's diabetes was clearly out of control, and he would readily agree about this. Sometimes we'd get off on how his life was stressful and made it hard for him to take care of himself, but most of the time he knew this was a flimsy excuse and he'd say so. I talked with him a lot about the medical dangers of where he was headed... told him about patients who had had amputations and all that... but things didn't really change. It occurred to me at one point to ask him what was the most important thing in his life. He said his daughter, who was then about two. I asked him to picture a time when he felt particularly close to his daughter. He described sitting on the sofa reading to her in the evening, with his daughter falling asleep in his arms. I asked Bob why this was important to him... I really knew the answer without asking... and he said that he just loved his daughter and wanted to give her the experience of having a good dad. We talked a little more about the connections between being a good dad and taking care of himself and diabetic outcomes... motivational interviewing stuff... and he's really been doing pretty well since that time.

As you probably know, the field of motivational interviewing forms some similar ideas into a clinical paradigm of exploring with people why they would want to remain the same and why they would want to change.[10] There are good data about the effectiveness of helping patients to sort through the reasons motivating their behavioral choices and to make choices that arise out of their personal values.

Life transitions

For all of us, transitions can be times for reflection and reappraisal. Changes like commitment to a partner, birth of a child, starting a new job, retirement, or deaths of parents transform the landscape of your life and present opportunities to envision the kind of person you want to be in your newly-configured roles.

Some of the most sacred times in my own life have been my marriage 36 years ago, the births of our three children, the passing of my parents in 1993 and 2000, and the marriage of our daughter to a bright and devoted man last year. If being father of the bride doesn't make you think about what's important in your life… walking down an aisle arm-in-arm with the child, now a woman, with whom you have shared birthday parties, bedtime stories, bike riding, school sports, travel around the country, proms, college visiting, and graduate school… nothing will.

With our patients, transitions can be good times for spiritual inquiry. As you are concluding by now, I don't think of this in terms of formal spiritual history-taking as much as just asking a conversational-language question that invites patients to reflect on "the vital and sacred" in their forthcoming roles. Examples:

- *What do you picture it like for you being a mom… what kind of mom do you hope to be?*
- *What prompts you to change to this new job? What is it, in particular, that is important to you that you hope will be better served in this new role?*
- *Last child leaving home… wow. How is that going to be for the two of you… what do you hope your relationship with Jeff will be like now that you're back to being more of a couple again?*
- *So sorry about your dad. I know how much you meant to each other and how devoted you have been taking care of him. I'm curious… where do you go from here? What do you see yourself putting energy into at this point as you try to adjust to his loss?*

With my particular style, I find that these types of questions about "What kind of person do you want to be?" and "How do you wish to be approaching this?" are often good entry points for spiritual inquiry. I can then follow up with more particular CAMPS questions *("So… what are some things that you are passionate about that you would hope to focus more on now that you are facing retirement?")* as situations warrant.

Bad news

Recall again our definition of spiritual care ("helping people to connect with the things that really matter to them") and that of palliative care and hospice consultant J. S. Lunn ("meeting people where they are and assisting them in connecting or reconnecting to things, practices, ideas, and principles that are at their core of their being.") These are particularly good frameworks for spiritual inquiry in the setting of "bad news."

Meeting people where they are means, first, recognizing and honoring the suffering that people bring. Several years ago, I met with the father of a young man who had been killed in a motor vehicle collision with a moose. Tragically, people die every year in Maine running into moose; they are twilight-colored and hard to see at a distance, they have no sense of roadways being human territory, and the bulk of their massive bodies is at windshield height. I recall the first conversation with this distraught man having little to do with meaning, purpose and spiritual sense-making; it really had to do much more with my attempt to just be a caring presence and to give him the opportunity to tell his story about the accident and about his son.

This is an essential first step in conversations with people about bad news… the bank teller who has been held up at gunpoint, the man who has just had a stroke at age 53, the woman who has just learned about a recurrence of ovarian cancer… being present to them with healing intention and creating the emotional and spiritual space for them to tell the stories they need to tell. Focusing on the noble questions of how people cope or where they find spiritual support before they feel heard and understood can be terribly dismissive.

As we meet people where they are, we move to the complementary piece of supporting people's meaningful connections… "connecting with the things that really matter," or "…assisting them in connecting or reconnecting to things, practices, ideas, and principles that are at their core of their being." The spiritual inquiry, therefore, involves:

- What are the "things, practices, ideas, and principles that are at their core of their being?"
- How are they doing with the "connecting or reconnecting?"
- What can they do to further strengthen their connections or re-connections with these things, going forward?

Clinician: *So the two of you have gotten over the initial shock of Melissa's breast cancer diagnosis and you have decided to go for the mastectomy. How would you put into words what's going to help you make your ways through this?*

Melissa: *We're in it together… I couldn't go through this without Steve.*

Steve: *Yea… that and our faith… we've kind of fallen away from church in the last few years, but we were talking about our faith always still being there and being important to us.*

Clinician: *Your caring for each other… great. When you mention "your faith," how is it that that is important to you right now?*

Steve: *God doesn't give you more than you can handle…*

Melissa: *That and the idea that everything happens for a reason.*

Clinician: *Is there some "reason" that you see at this point?*

Melissa: *I don't know… maybe it'll make us closer… I guess it has done that… maybe it'll bring us back to church.*

Steve: *Closer, yea… but I'm still kind of burned out on church… for me, the main thing is just trusting God together to work this out.*

This brief spiritual inquiry has established a number of points. Caring for each other is sustaining for this couple, and they hope that Melissa's illness may bring them closer together. "Faith" is important to them, not so much in the form of institutional connections, as privately. The ideas that things happen for a reason and that God will be working things out are parts of their belief system, although just what they might mean at this point is not completely clear.

Spiritual struggles and issues

Much of our exploration in this chapter has focused on spiritual resources; identifying and encouraging people in the expression of values and practices that lend meaning and spiritual vitality to their lives. What about the "spiritual issues" side? What do you say to people who are furious at God for allowing egregious suffering... the 29 year old mother of two infant children who has just been diagnosed with end-stage breast cancer, or the parents of a beautiful young child who has been disfigured in a fire? What do you say to people who are locked into spiritual desperation or hopelessness... like the aging man who feels estranged from his faith and is increasingly despondent that he may never be able to heal a decades-long rift with his son? What does "spiritual inquiry" consist of in the setting of suffering like this?

Fundamentally, it is the same. The same paradigm applies; meeting people where they are, understanding what has been meaningful in their lives, and inviting them to connect or re-connect with those sources of meaning and spiritual vitality.

The pace may be very different, however. As with the example of the father of the moose collision victim, the pace moves slowly. People need to experience a caring presence and to be honored in being able to tell their stories. It is, as I have suggested before, excellent spiritual care just to be present to people in this way.

Even as we affirm where people are, however, all of us as clinicians would want to encourage people in moving beyond their pain and suffering.

Tempting as it may be, telling people the "right" answer from our own life experience is rarely helpful in these situations. "God knows what He is doing and this will all turn out to His glory." "Come, come... your having had the affair didn't cause you to have cancer... God doesn't punish people like that... these things just happen." "You just have to let it go with your son... you've done the best that you can." Maybe there are some clinicians out there who are wiser than I am and who can present opinions like this in a convincing way... but my experience is that people need to come to their own truth.

Spiritual care in situations like these... and here, "inquiry" merges with "intervention," as we have discussed... is much more "asking" than "telling." Spiritual inquiry in situations like these, I believe, means gently opening up the possibility of a future that is somehow more coherent and that could make sense.

- *"Wow, I can imagine how any loving parent would be devastated... and probably furious... about something like this. How in the world do parents come to grips with this?"*
- *"Doubts about your faith and the pain around your son... how have you managed to live with this... what has kept you going so far?"*
- *"You agree with your mom that you need to forgive yourself but this really is a whole lot easier said than done, isn't it? A great question... how do people somehow make peace with the bad choices that they have made?"*

None of these questions presents or prescribes a solution, but they frame the issue. They focus the conversation on the possibility of a different outcome. We will explore pathways to solutions extensively in the next chapter.

Painful and unremitting suffering in cases like these often also calls for the involvement and partnership of our spiritual care specialist colleagues. The end point of the conversation with health care clinicians is often, appropriately, "I have a chaplain colleague who is really helpful with people sorting out struggles like this," or "Who is there out there that you trust who can help you to work through the spiritual issues that you are raising?"

STRATEGY 12
Adapt spiritual inquiry to the circumstances where you see people

Consider the circumstances we have explored... well person visits, lifestyle change, life transitions, bad news, and spiritual struggles and issues. Reflect on which among these would be the areas that would most merit more cogent spiritual inquiry in your practice. Adapt the questions you have developed in Strategy 11 to these circumstances.

FINAL WORDS

When I distribute the CAMPS sidebar to groups in workshops, I have several bullets at the bottom that offer as reminders of some important perspectives to carry with us as we pursue spiritual inquiry. We have considered several of these issues in the chapter, but I want to list them here for emphasis. They are:

- Use conversational (not spirituo-jargonoid) language that is comfortable for you.
- Inquire in the context of
  o the PAST ("When have there been times...")
  o the PRESENT ("How do you...")
  o the FUTURE ("How do you hope that, as you go along...")
- Be alert to cues from patients... picking up on cues is as (or more) important than asking cold questions.
- Ask patients pertinent questions and invite them to think about answers. Their wisdom counts more than our wisdom.
- Bear in mind the critical importance of *genuineness of spirit* in these inquiries. "Intention" is more important than clock time.
- Be charitable with yourself...you can't do it all, all the time.

SUMMARY

- Spiritual inquiry and spiritual intervention are typically woven together in a fluid process. With some exceptions (such as integrative medicine consultation), they are not sequential.
- Spiritual inquiry is pursued with inventories and in conversation. Inventories are well constructed, but typically are suited for research purposes more than clinical purposes.
- Three conversational templates for formal spiritual inquiry... the SPIRITual history, HOPE and FICA... offer helpful structures for conversation.
- The CAMPS template offers a practical framework of dimensions of spiritual experience, along with questions for exploration.
- Some recommendations for spiritual inquiry with CAMPS include:
  o Picking and choosing questions that fit for you.
  o Picking up on patients' experience and cues as much as possible
  o Using conversational language and using patients' language for their own spiritual beliefs and experience
- Think of spiritual inquiry in the settings of
  o Well person visits
  o Lifestyle change
  o Life transitions
  o Bad news
  o Spiritual struggles and issues

REFERENCES

1. Carson V, Koenig H. *Spiritual Caregiving: Health Care as a Ministry.* West Conshohocken, PA: Templeton Foundation Press; 2004.
2. Peterman AH, Fitchett G, Brady MJ, Hernandez L, Cella D. Measuring spiritual well-being in people with cancer: The Functional Assessment of Chronic Illness Therapy- Spiritual Well-Being Scale (FACIT-Sp). *Annals of Beh Med.* 2002;24(1):49-58.

3. Dailey D, Stewart A. Psychometric characteristics of the spiritual perspective scale in pregnant African-American women. *Res Nurs Health.* 2007;30(1):61-71.

4. VandeCreek L, Ayres S, Bassham M. Using INSPIRIT to conduct spiritual assessments. *J Pastoral Care.* Spring 1995;49(1):83-89.

5. Kass J. Self-test for our "age of anxiety". *Spirituality and Health.* 2003(November/December):56-59.

6. Maugans TA. The SPIRITual history. *Arch Fam Med.* Jan 1996;5(1):11-16.

7. Anandarajah G, Hight E. Spirituality and medical practice: Using the HOPE questions as a practical tool for spiritual assessment. *Am Fam Physician.* Jan 1 2001;63(1):81-89.

8. Puchalski CM. Taking a spiritual history: FICA. *Spirituality and medicine connection.* 1999;3(1):1.

9. Ewing J. Detecting alcoholism. The CAGE questionnaire. *JAMA.* 1984;252(14):1905-1907.

10. Miller W, Rollnick S, Conforti K. *Motivational Interviewing: Preparing People for Change.* New York: Guilford; 2002.

Chapter Nine

Partner with Patients in Pursuing What They Care About

Real change begins with the simple act
of people talking about what they care about.[1]

Margaret Wheatley

We discussed in the last chapter the idea that inquiry and intervention are joined together in a fluid process. Curiosity about another person goes along with the hope for a brighter future, and the *process of inquiry* about what has been and is important moves people in the *direction* of what is important.

An internist recounts:

I have students rotate through my office and I usually give them the first shot at working with patients, with my supervision. A student was seeing a diabetic woman with me and the conversation turned to her smoking. The student did what I presume he had been taught to do... told her about all of the health effects of smoking, black lungs, feet falling off. He asked her if she thought she should stop and she said "yes" in a somewhat hesitant, drawn-out way. He then gave her a sincere but somewhat disjointed set of instructions about keeping track of her cigarettes, how much she wanted to smoke each one, cutting out the easy ones first and then setting a quit date. Told her to have a supply of carrot sticks to help with the urge to hold something. "Any questions," he asked. The poor woman looked pretty bewildered but didn't have any questions. She didn't strike me as a carrot stick kind of person.

I asked her a few motivational interviewing questions... what was good about smoking (it helped her to relax) and what was not so good (she knew the health issues backwards and forwards). I asked her how much she wanted to quit and why... she said she did want to quit and the main thing for her was being able to follow her grandchildren around. Then I asked if she had ever quit before. Yes, she had, once for seven or eight years. How did she do that? She brightened as she spoke about it... she said she just "remembered her spirituality." What did this mean? She said she would just get up each morning and remember that God had a plan for her life. When she got the urge to smoke, she just "turned it over." We talked about this for a couple more minutes... she said she had been thinking that she had gotten away from her spirituality... and she left I think with some confidence that she could pull it off again. The student and I had a good conversation afterwards, essentially about the idea that the first thing you do is find out what motivates people to change and how they have managed to change before.

This is good spiritual care. The internist supports this patient in connecting to what is vital and sacred in her life. The patient is helped to reconnect to her vision of interacting meaningfully with her grandchildren, with the personal foundation of her spirituality, and with God's plans for her life.

I would not particularly call this conversation "counseling" (although we might have to use that word for billing purposes). When we think of spiritual care conversations like this as "counseling," it conjures up too much the specialty care model we discussed in Chapter 1, with the attendant feelings of weariness at the prospect of somehow needing to learn sophisticated and specialized skills.

"Counseling," after all, has its roots in the process of giving advice. You know by now that I love word origins. Our modern word "counsel" comes from the Latin "consilium," meaning "plan," or "opinion." The medical student presented plans and opinions; the internist did not.

Rather than advice-giving, the approach of the internist was collaborative. It was exploration together with the patient of what mattered to her. The solution, in this conversation, arose primarily out of the wisdom and life experience of the patient.

There is nothing inherently wrong with advice-giving in health and wellness care. Indeed, we all have training and expertise that allows us to help patients precisely because we can give advice. I know the empirical literature on behavioral approaches to anxiety and depression. You perhaps know the empirical literature on pharmacological, or integrative medicine approaches to anxiety and depression. You may have expertise in the Western health care treatment of hypertension, osteoporosis, or irritable bowel syndrome. You may be an expert about nutritional issues. You may practice Chinese medicine and have a wealth of knowledge and experience in treating conditions that have no Western equivalents whatsoever.

This knowledge and experience that we bring to patients is often vitally important. In the realm of spiritual care, however… anchored in the journey toward what is "vital and sacred" for people and what "really matters" to them… the conversation has to welcome the values, goals, life experiences, and wisdom that patients bring.

Spiritual care conversations are a partnership. They are collaborative. You and I have wisdom and patients have wisdom. The wisdom that we all bring is directed toward patients' goals, patients' values, and toward what helps patients to be spiritually alive and whole.

In this chapter, I want to consider with you some practical approaches to spiritual care conversations in partnership with patients. In the next chapter, we will look at some recurring themes in these conversations, such as mindfulness, serenity, forgiveness, and valued directions.

A TEMPLATE FOR COLLABORATIVE SPIRITUAL CARE CONVERSATIONS

Having a structure or framework for organizing what we are doing guides the directions we pursue and the choices we make. As Yogi says, if you don't know where you're going, you're probably not going to get there.

In health care, we have abundant templates and algorithms to guide us in choosing particular treatments. There are good algorithms for when you get someone going on C-pap, when you prescribe hydrochlorothiazide, when you do desensitization, and when you administer moxibustion.

In the venue of integrative medicine where I have taught for a number of years, clinicians thoroughly review someone's history and presentation and then propose a multifaceted treatment plan. The elements of the treatment plans are, for the most part, specific interventions. An integrative medicine clinician might propose a nutritional program, a botanical treatment, a mind-body approach, some form of energy medicine, or Qigong.

We do *not* so much have templates in health care at the level of our *conversations* with patients. Some time ago, I recall observing a new intern… a recent medical school graduate… having a counseling session with a patient. The apparent strategy was to get the patient talking about what troubled her and to ask repeatedly, "How do you feel about that?" This seemed to be the template for the conversation… "Get them talking about troubles and get them to describe their feelings." It was not apparent that the intern had any plan for what she would do as people express their feelings. In fairness, I suspect that there was no attention at all in her medical school to working with patients at the level of conversations; she came fairly well versed in pharmacological treatments for DSM diagnoses, but not in approaches to talking with people. This young woman, by the way, turned out to be an outstanding physician.

Spiritual care, in particular, is less a matter of recommending specific interventions… although it can be that… than it is being intentional about how we talk with people. There are specific spiritual care interventions, as we have discussed… meditation, prayer, gratefulness approaches, chaplain consultation, and so forth… but the foundation of spiritual care is being present to people, understanding their values, and being partners on their journeys.

A template for collaborative spiritual care conversations

Three elements and some samples of conversation

Presuming a background of trust and patients feeling valued and understood…

1. Where do you want to go?

   What do you care about?
   What is your goal?
   What do you wish to accomplish?
   How would you like to be different?
   How would you like to be handling this?
   What kind of person do you want to be as you move through this?

2. How are you going to get there?

   a. Your (patient's) wisdom

   What is your sense about what you do now?
   When are the times when you feel like you're moving forward?
   What have you learned in your life that applies to this?

   b. My (clinician's) wisdom

   This is what the data say.
   This is what my patients have said.
   This is what I have learned from my experience.

3. What is the next step?

   What will you do to follow up at this point?
   What do you see yourself putting energy into now?
   When we next meet, what would you hope to report?

The sidebar presents a template for spiritual care conversations. The template presumes that patients feel respected and understood.

Some time ago, I spoke with a practice manager at a specialty clinic who was interested in developing a spiritual screening program. The draft proposal was that an intake worker would ask patients whether spirituality provided a source of strength and comfort to them. This particular question... whether people find strength and comfort from spirituality... is indeed prominent in the spirituality and health literature. But having an intake worker ask this question... absent of any substantial relationship with patients, alongside questions about diarrhea yes-or-no and insurance policy number... will not work. This is a question that needs to arise from a foundation of trust and healing intention.

The first element of the template is ***where people want to go.*** Defining how people want to be, or want to change, helps to establish a shared goal and a spirit of partnership. The second element is ***how people are going to get there.*** This brings together patients' wisdom from life experience and intuition, and clinicians' wisdom from empirical data, patient experiences, and personal experience as professionals and as human beings.

The final element is identifying ***next steps.*** I am firmly persuaded that people who leave health care visits and do something concrete to follow up have better outcomes than those who do not. It seems to me, moreover, that the specifics of what people do to follow up is less important than *that* they do something to follow up.

Let's look at these elements of the conversational template in greater detail.

GOALS: WHAT MATTERS TO YOU AND WHERE DO YOU WANT TO GO?

Collaborative spiritual care conversions are anchored in a definition of the goal. People often come to us with the mindset that they will tell us what is wrong with their lives, medically and psychosocially. It is, of course, vital to listen to and honor what patients tell us about what is wrong. It is equally important, however, to help patients move beyond the conversation about what is wrong and to put into words what the goal is and where they want to be going.

Future vision… patients creating a definition or image of where they want to be going… provides direction and energy, and provides a positive anchor point for our conversations with them about coping and health behavior choices.

Someone challenged by anxiety or depression: How do they want their life to be different? Someone having a hard time with diabetic control: How do they want their approach to diabetes to be different from what it is now? Someone complaining of chronic pain: What would they hope to be doing differently if they were coping with pain better?

Some examples of conversation starters that begin to explore where patients want to go:

- *What is your goal?*
- *What do you wish to accomplish?*
- *How would you like to be handling this?*
- *What do you hope for?*
- *What kind of person do you want to be as you move through this?*
- *What, in particular, really matters to you about this?*
- *How do you want your life to be different?*
- *Six months from now, what will we be seeing about how you have moved forward with this?*
- *What would I notice about you if you were a little more on top of things?*

As we think about goals and conversation starters, I particularly want to commend the quotation that begins this chapter. Margaret Wheatley is an organizational consultant who writes for an organizational development audience as well as for a broader audience of people interested in change and partnership in wider social systems. "Real change," she says, "begins with the simple act of people talking about what they care about."[1] Real change… not superficial or transient, but real change… begins with the simple act of people talking about what they care about. What matters to them. What is vitally important to them.

When you talk about what you care about, there is very different energy compared with talking about more pedestrian topics. An applicant to our residency program a couple of weeks ago was dutifully articulate in speaking with me about some of the philosophical underpinnings of family medicine. She really lit up, though, when she spoke about working in a free clinic in inner city Cleveland and about the richness in human experience and caring in which she took part there. She *agrees* with the philosophical underpinnings; she is *engaged with her heart* in having caring relationships with underserved people.

Getting people talking about what they care about… I often suggest at workshops that this is a great foundation for spiritual care.

There are a number of important principles as we consider approaches to exploring patients' goals.

Goals can be outcomes or values

You will see, from the above list, that "where you want to go" may be framed in terms of outcomes or values. **Outcomes** are typically specific, functional end points. A woman wishes to decide whether she should leave an abusive relationship. A cancer patient wants to complete a notebook for grown children. Someone who says they have been struggling for years with chronic fatigue syndrome wants to be more selective about saying "yes" or "no" to commitments. A man with chronic pain wants to get to the point of spending more time away from his home.

Values often pertain to qualities of character, as we considered in Chapter 6. The abused woman wishes to "be strong" and to "show the importance of courage and determination" to her children. The cancer patient wants to "maintain his dignity" and to "be thankful." The person with fatigue wants to "think of myself as being as important as other people." The man with chronic pain wants to "not give up and keep pushing."

Goals in spiritual care conversations are rooted in the "vital and sacred"

Collaborative goals in spiritual care conversations are grounded in things that really matter to people. For both outcomes and values, goals that relate to what is "vital and sacred" in people's lives are qualitatively different from changes people may wish to make that are more specific or prosaic. Goals relating to what is vital and sacred have very different energy from more concrete ideas or plans for change. Consider:

I think I will take up stamp collecting again.

For most of us, this is not a particularly inspiring or energizing goal. I did have a friend once whose fondest dream was finding one of those upside-down airplane stamps in an old trunk, but this would not excite most people. By itself, the prospect of resuming stamp collecting might be a perfectly fine change someone would wish to make, but is not a particularly meaningful goal in the context of spiritual care. Consider, however:

The oncologist says that most people at Stage IV are done for in a few months. This absolutely sucks… but what am I going to do… give up and just go away? Maybe it won't be too long, but I really have to keep living my life.

"Keep living my life" in the setting of end-stage cancer is a pretty good goal. It certainly touches on qualities of determination and perseverance that probably define who this person is. If this person decided that a good way to keep living his life would be to take up stamp collecting again, the idea of stamp collecting again feels very different. It is a specific methodology in service of a personally meaningful goal, and some of the spirit of sacredness of the goal of "living my life" rubs off.

As you see in the template we are considering, I think that a definition of both spiritually-meaningful goals and of concrete steps is important. The conversation can flow in either direction.

Patient: *I think I'll take up stamp collecting again.*
Clinician: *OK... how would you put into words why that is important for you right now?*
Patient: *I have to keep living my life.*

or

Patient: *I have to keep living my life.*
Clinician: *OK... give me an example of how you see yourself doing that right now.*
Patient: *I think I'll take up stamp collecting again.*

In inquiring about spiritually-meaningful goals, we help patients by orienting their thoughts and hearts to the core values that they cherish.

Affirming and, in a sense, expressing solidarity with people's values, moreover, are central parts of spiritual care. In the Ronald Reagan assassination attempt, the president was conscious and alert as he was removed from the scene and taken by ambulance to the hospital. Being wheeled into the surgical suite and introduced to the surgeon, Reagan flashed his noted sense of humor, telling the surgeon that he hoped he was a Republican. The surgeon replied, "Today, sir, we are all Republicans." We may or may not share the particular values that other people have, but we can honor the importance of the core values in their lives.

Clinician: *So it's looking like the tests are reassuring about the cancer... how are you doing with this... how are you doing emotionally?*
Patient: *It's good to hear, but I still get really keyed up.*
Clinician [asking how she would wish to be, "instead"]: *Keyed up... OK... how would you hope to be as you go through this instead of keyed up?*
Patient: *I just need to relax, stop thinking as much and just get a better grip or perspective on things.*
Clinician [exploring the values behind what the patient is saying]: *Could you say a little more about why in particular it would be important for you to relax and stop thinking and get a grip?*

Patient: *Apart from the fact that I'm driving myself nuts, it really isn't fair to my husband and children to be so preoccupied... or distracted.*
Clinician: *You want to be there more for your family...*
Patient: *Yea, doing everything I can to create a good home for my family...*
Clinician [affirming the patient's values and exploring how her stated goals might be manifest]: *I can see how important that is to you. So when you say "relax, stop thinking as much and get a better perspective," say more about what that looks like...*

Goals are within patients' control

We can really only join with patients on goals that are attainable, and the circumstances that come at us are not always changeable. Many of the circumstances that I talk with people about involve the behavior of other people... partners, supervisors, children, neighbors... and it may or may not be productive to explore goals and approaches to get the other people to change their behavior. Similarly, the course of illnesses may sometimes be changeable, and sometimes are likely not to be changeable.

Patient, six months after stroke: *It's still really frustrating... I can't remember things like I used to... I can't find words like I always have been able to do... I'm really tired of people asking me how I'm doing with that sympathetic look all the time.*
Clinician [expressing empathy, sounding out likelihood that circumstances can change]: *I can imagine. What does your neurologist say about where things are likely to go from here?*
Patient: *She doesn't know... it could get better, it could stay the same forever.*
Clinician [acknowledging uncertain course of stroke effects, inviting patient to turn attention to how he wants to be living with this uncertainty]: *Actually, that's what I'd say, too. Wow... how does somebody deal with that uncertainty... so how would you hope to be handling this for however long it's hanging over your head?*

Patient: *What can I do... just do the best I can.*
Clinician [looking for behavioral reference points that can help in defining goals and approaches]: *OK... good... and what does that consist of, for you... "doing the best you can?"*

Often, a screening question like *"To what extent do you think this is something that you can change, that you can be making different?"* gives a clear indication about whether there could be a productive conversation about changing circumstances. Sometimes, patients will answer this question... particularly when the presenting circumstances involve dissatisfaction about the behavior of somebody else... with a resounding "NO... THEY'LL NEVER CHANGE!" In such cases, it is good to get this reality out on the table earlier rather than later.

Sometimes there may be a difference of perspective between clinicians and patients about the possibility of changing circumstances. Perhaps your patient with metastatic pancreatic cancer retains hope for a miraculous cure. I would not want to take this hope away, and at the same time I would want to gently turn the conversation toward living with dignity for whatever time remains.

Developing collaborative goals about changing internal experiences like thoughts, feelings and somatic sensations can be particularly challenging. The pharmaceutical industry reinforces...or has perhaps created...the cultural presumption that distressing personal experiences can be summarily dispatched with pills. Sleep problems? Erectile dysfunction? Restless legs? Gas? Social anxiety disorder? Pain? Take a pill and you won't even need to call me in the morning.

With many of these internal experiences, though, the harder you try to control them, the more powerful they become. The harder you try not to be anxious, to go to sleep, or to put worrisome thoughts out of your mind, the more these experiences tend to persist and grow. In the next chapter, we will explore approaches to helping people to live with circumstances that are not controllable and changeable.

Overall, the premise that goals in spiritual care conversations need to be within patients' control often moves the conversations toward qualities of character... as we discussed in Chapter 6. You may or may not be able to control the circumstances that come at you or the ways that the world reacts to you, but you can always choose whether or not to be kind... or grateful... or curious... or persevering.

Goals in spiritual care conversations are positively framed

People can frame goals in terms of doing less of what they don't want to do, or in terms of doing more of what matters to them. Go with the latter.

Maybe I need to be less cynical.

or

I want to be more generous.

Even though there is probably some conceptual overlap between these two statements of goals, framing the goal as becoming more generous is preferable to framing the goal as being less cynical. First, the technology or methodology of establishing behavior patterns is more substantial than the technology or methodology of diminishing behavior patterns. I'll bet you can think of twelve ways to be more generous more quickly than twelve ways to be less cynical.

Second, a conversation around positive goals has very different energy than conversations around diminishing problems. When I meet with couples in my practice, for instance, conversations around how they can understand and support each other is consistently more energizing and hopeful than conversations around how they could fight and argue less.

Strategically, the key word is "instead."

Clinician: *Hey, look at your date of birth... you're going to be 50 next Tuesday... congratulations.*

Patient: *I'm not sure what 50 is supposed to feel like, but I don't think I feel 50.*

Clinician: *Good for you. When you look back on the last 50 years and look forward to the next 50… what do you see yourself focusing on in the years to come?*

Patient: *I think I've got to stop taking life so seriously.*

Clinician: *How do you mean?*

Patient: *I don't know… I think I always make a big deal out of things… I worry too much.*

Clinician: *OK… how would you wish to be instead of taking life too seriously?*

Patient: *Just take it as it comes.*

Clinician: *Sounds good… tell me more about that…*

The "instead" moves the conversation in the opposite direction. The clinician can explore what "take it as it comes" means to this person, and what this person can do to move more in that direction.

So it can be with any negatively-framed experience:

less depressed	>	more active
less anxious	>	more confident
less angry	>	more patient or understanding
less limited by pain	>	more functional in spite of pain
less preoccupation with illness	>	more engagement with things that matter

Goals in spiritual care conversations use patients' language

I often find it very helpful to look for or elicit patients' language for where they want to be going. I ask "How would you "put into words…"

- *What you would like to accomplish?"*
- *How you would like to change?"*

- *How you would like to be different?"*
- *What would tell us that you are moving forward?"*

...and I pay close attention to the language they use in what they say.

In the last week, people have answered these questions...

- *I want to figure out "who Donna really is."*
- *I want to separate myself from my children's problems.*
- *I need to stay in the present time.*
- *I think I can handle all of this as long as I concentrate on doing the right thing.*
- *I need to work on bettering myself.*

Let me point out, by the way, that these are not cream-off-the-top, articulate, college-educated, existentially-oriented intellectuals; they are regular folk who are putting into words what they want for their lives.

When people say things like this, I pay attention and I frequently anchor conversations in their language. I do this for two reasons. First, patients' language has richness of meaning and information. I don't have any idea what "who Donna is" means or what "doing the right thing" means, but patients do, and they are saying this because it matters to them. Second, there is a very different energy in orienting conversations to what is meaningful for patients rather than what is meaningful to me. "How are you doing with your effort to better yourself?" has very different energy than "How are you doing with your bipolar disorder NOS?"

The principle of using patients' language in spiritual care conversations is particularly important for language that is expressly spiritual. References to the experience of spirituality ("my spirituality," "my faith," "my practices") and to a superordinate presence or deity ("God," "Buddha," "Spirit," "the Universe," "the Man Upstairs") needs to be in language that comes from patients.

Goals may be directed toward three choices

People come to us in distress about challenging life circumstances. These may be external (such as financial hardships or other people's behavior) or internal (such as physical symptoms or medical illnesses, troublesome emotions, and troublesome thoughts). People have three choices in dealing with distressing life circumstances.

1. Changing the circumstances.
2. Coping with the circumstances.
3. Being healthy and whole in spite of whatever is going on with distressing circumstances.

Changing the circumstances. Sometimes people can be invited to define goals and encouraged to do problem-solving that could potentially change the circumstances that they face. In a sense, this is the main work of what we do in the day to day business of health care. People look to us to remove cancerous lesions, to repair torn ACLs, to collaborate with them in lowering cholesterol, or reducing the frequency of headaches. We can certainly also join with patients on meaningful goals for changing health-related circumstances that are not specifically medical, such as getting organized financially, repairing an alienated relationship with a parent, or deciding whether or not to move to that retirement community in Bullhead City.

As we considered above, the key question for goals about changing circumstances is whether this is plausible. Healing a fractured wrist with a program of splinting is possible; healing the pain of abuse by getting the perpetrator to beg for forgiveness may not be plausible.

Coping with the circumstances. The second choice in dealing with distressing life circumstances… around which we may collaborate with patients on goals… has to do with coping.

People may not have choices about the circumstances of their lives, but they do have choices about their reactions to those circumstances. When people present with painful or ambiguous situations

Three choices in relating to life circumstances

1. Change the circumstances

   - Change the reality
       i. out there (e.g., finances, housing, behavior of other people)
       ii. in there (e.g., medical, surgical, self-care treatment of illness)
   - Leave

2. Cope with the circumstances

   - Change attitudes (e.g., mindfulness instead of victimization)
   - Change behaviors (e.g., kindness instead of belligerence)

3. Be healthy and whole in spite of circumstances

   - Nutrition
   - Exercise
   - Passions, fun
   - Learning and growing
   - Social connections
   - Expression of personal values
   - Connections with Spirit

that are not clearly within their control, I often ask, *"How are you coping with this?* or *"How are you handling this?"*

For me, this comes up in two settings.

- Expressing compassion and turning the conversation to how people are handling medical problems, while they are pursuing appropriate care

So you're working with your oncologist on the cancer... how are you doing with all of this... how are you coping with all of this?

- Reinforcing people's abilities to make choices and exploring how people *wish to be* coping with circumstances

Patient: *I wasn't surprised that I'd have a flare-up of my Crohn's disease... it's been incredibly stressful at work.*
Clinician: *We've talked about the flare-up... how do you see yourself coping with the stress at work?*

Patient: *There's not much I can do... much too much work, people out on medical leave which just makes more work for the rest of us... a supervisor who is on everybody's case and just makes it worse...*

Clinician: *Wow... is it your sense that there are things you can do to change this environment?*

Patient: *Fire the supervisor and hire twelve new people.*

Clinician: *I'll take that as a "no."*

Patient: *For sure.*

Clinician: *So if things aren't destined to change soon in your workplace, what is your sense about what you can do to make the best of it... to cope with it?*

Patient: *I don't know... I have been trying to take my breaks recently and making a point not to work through lunch... I think that helps some...*

Clinician: *Good. What else?*

Patient: *Um...*

Clinician: *Let me ask you what will feel like a silly question... if you set out to conduct yourself at work in order to make the stress get to you as much as you can, what would you do?*

Patient: *Sit at my desk and read Soap Opera Digest all day.*

Clinician: *I like your sense of humor... humor is healing.*

Patient: *I would join in the "this sucks" conversation with my co-workers at every opportunity.*

Clinician: *Good. And do you do this?*

Patient: *No, I've also been thinking recently that this really drags me down and this isn't really the kind of person I want to be... so I have been laying off.*

Clinician: *What difference does that make for you?*

Patient: *I think I'm a little more balanced... I usually try to be someone who brings calm into the world and it feels good to be that way a little more.*

Clinician: *Cool. You're describing a couple of good examples of ways that you try to cope with a pretty tough situation... giving yourself a break and being the person that you want to be. How would you put*

into words how you would want to be coping in your workplace in the next few months?
Patient: *Balanced, I guess... more balance.*

You will notice, by the way, that neither of the last two interview transcript examples contains the word "spirituality." They do, however, touch on personal values and qualities that are meaningful for these people. The stroke victim speaks of "doing the best he can." The woman with Crohn's disease speaks about "balance" and being someone who "brings calm into the world." Spiritual care is not an enterprise that necessarily involves spiritual or specialty language... it does involve the common-sense process of meeting people where they are and helping them to connect to things that matter to them.

Being healthy and whole in spite of whatever is going on with distressing circumstances. The third choice in dealing with distressing life circumstances... around which we may collaborate with patients on goals... has to do with the choices people make about healthy and meaningful living apart from whatever ways they may seek to deal with the challenges that come their way. We can support and encourage people to live in health-enhancing and meaningful ways as they go along... like eating right, exercising, finding some pleasure and joy, learning something new, caring about the people that they love, and making choices about how they spend their time and energy consistent with their values.

In my practice, I suspect that I recommend exercise and fun as much as anything else. Exercise... such as walking, swimming, gym equipment, biking, and my own favorite of 25 years, basketball... unclog your arteries, tone your muscles, connect you with other people, and give you a sense of accomplishment. Fun, similarly, has a way of restoring the soul. I think that we culturally value fun... with its attendant joy and laughter... too little. For a number of years, I have made a point of asking patients (as well as colleagues and friends) what they do for fun. To my dismay, the most frequent answers I get are "Nothing," "Are you kidding" and "I don't have much time for fun."

The Resilience table from Chapter 7 touches on a number of areas about healthy and meaningful living. We can also encourage people in goals around spiritual life and growth, along the lines of the dimensions of spirituality reflected in the CAMPS questions.

Goals in spiritual care conversations move patients beyond complaints

Finally, let me suggest a couple of specific phrases that I find useful in making the transition in these conversations between complaints and goals.

- *What are you trying to figure out?*

or

- *What questions are you trying to answer with this that we can work on together?*

People bring to us all sorts of troubles. The patient says "I'm really depressed." Now the ball is in your court to say or propose something wise that will fix them. Asking *what they are trying to figure out* puts the ball back in *their* court; it moves patients into a position where they take some responsibility for organizing the conversation around where they want to go with the symptoms they are giving you.

What I am looking for is a question from patients along the lines of "How do I..." Examples:

"Well, what can I do to get less depressed?"

"How do I deal with this?"

It is not hard to have patients state questions like these, and as they do, it moves them into the first step in taking ownership of the search for solutions.

An additional phrase that I find useful in making the transition in these conversations between complaints and goals:

"Hm... interesting question... how do you..."

With this question, I am in effect proposing a possible answer to "where do you want to go?" I am trying to bring together a variety of concerns the patient is expressing into a clearly-framed question that I believe could be fruitful for the patient to explore.

A 56 year old woman has presented with complaints of fatigue, which have been evaluated medically with no clear etiology. The conversation has turned to her history of emotional abandonment as a child, abuse from a former partner, and alienation from a woman who until recently was her best friend. The clinician (in a spirit of wondering out loud) asks,

"Wow, interesting question... so how does someone deal with this kind of pain in so many important relationships?

As with the question of what someone is trying to figure out, this approach can focus people's concerns or complaints in the direction of the question, "How do I...?" When people are at the point of asking this question (such as "Yea, how do I get over this kind of pain?"), they have formed a good goal and it also moves them a step toward taking ownership of the search for solutions.

STRATEGY 13: Get patients talking about what they care about

Particularly with patients who are challenging for you, spend a little time getting to know what matters to them and what they want. Experiment with the conversation-starter questions and find a way that fits for you of understanding where people want to be going.

APPROACHES: HOW ARE
YOU GOING TO GET THERE?

The first element in spiritual care conversations has to do with defining with patients where they wish to be going. The second element has to do with defining how they are going to get there.

This is, as I have said, a collaborative process. The conversation about solutions brings together *patients'* wisdom from life experience and intuition, and *clinicians'* wisdom from empirical data, patient experiences, and personal experience as professionals and as human beings.

Between the two…patients' wisdom and our wisdom… I believe that patients' wisdom holds particular value. As clinicians, we may have expertise in how people in general make changes and pursue health, but patients are experts on themselves. Their wisdom… how they have coped, how they have made changes, how they have pursued values that are meaningful for them… is important because it is specific to their lives ands because they own it.

Wisdom from patients

Consider first some ways that we may solicit ideas about "how are you going to get there" that arise from patients' wisdom and experience.

Catch patients in the act of being competent. Whenever patients report some accomplishment… stopping drinking, logging blood pressures, making dietary changes, handling a motor vehicle accident with some degree of grace… I like to acknowledge that and, if possible, talk about how and why they did it. All of us instinctively try to be enthusiastic about patients' efforts. In addition to this, I think that the "how" and "why" questions can often reinforce people's competence.

"No alcohol for 5 years… wow. How did you do that?"

"It's striking to me that you have had this profound accident and here you are in a wheelchair, but you're still pretty cheerful... what is this like for you and how do you do it?"

"You say you have been working on your diet... what changes have you been making, in particular?"

"You're telling me you're pretty burned out, but you're still going to work and taking care of your kids... what keeps you holding it together as much as you are?"

There are three reasons for having these conversations with people, even briefly.

1. It is affirming for patients to have their clinicians recognize their efforts.
2. It gives us a window on how people individually cope with life.
3. It is more fun than talking about people's failures.

I find that many opportunities to catch people being competent come up in passing, in comments that people make that could easily pass by unless we are attuned to hearing them. The cues that I try to be attentive to are a) when people report having started some meaningful behavior pattern, and b) when people report or imply having stopped some behavior pattern that was good to have changed. Example:

Scenario #1:

Clinician, taking history: *So how did you do in school?*
Patient: *Not so great... I was pretty messed up as a kid.*
Clinician: *"Messed up?"*
Patient: *Yea, drugs, missed a lot of school...*
Clinician: *Did you graduate?*
Patient: *Well, I got a GED.*
Clinician: *And what do you do for work now?*

Scenario #2

Clinician, taking history: *So how did you do in school?*
Patient: *Not so great... I was pretty messed up as a kid.*
Clinician: *"Messed up?"*
Patient: *Yea, drugs, missed a lot of school...*
Clinician: *OK... you say "messed up as a kid..." so you stopped messing up at some point?*
Patient: *Yea, it took a few years but I think I pulled it together pretty well.*
Clinician: *So when did you pull it together and how did you do that?*
Patient: *I think it started when my dad died... he was killed in a forklift accident at work when I was 20... 21.*
Clinician: *Oh... sorry to hear... how did that affect you?*
Patient: *It really shook me up. I was... like I said, messed up... but I was close to my dad and I think it made me come to my senses and realize that you never know when your time's up and you've got to do something with your life.*
Clinician: *When you say "Do something with your life," say more about what that means to you...*

The first example is acceptable routine care. The second example catches the patient being competent. The clinician picks up on the presumption of past tense in the phrase, "when I was a kid" and inquires about how the patient stopped "messing up." The patient's answer... as is typically the case with explanations of significant life changes... points to a meaningful personal value, "doing something with your life."

Catching this patient being competent and eliciting this life value is good spiritual care and is important for several reasons. First, it is affirming for the patient. Second, it gives the clinician significant information that relates to the patient's health. By the patient's own account, "doing something with your life" had the significant health benefit of helping him to turn his life around.

Given the spirituality and health literature that we have reviewed, it is not much of a stretch to presume that the extent to which the patient "does something with his life" will play a significant role in his health and well-being going forward.

Third, it points to a direction of conversation that can address the question of "how are you going to get there?" The next exchange in the second scenario will do just that… exploring with the patient the specific methodology for doing something with life. Caring about other people, setting a good example for a child, making a difference in one's community… whatever the patient says in providing examples of "doing something with life," the clinician can encourage the patient in these particular approaches going forward.

Finally, hearing the story of how this person changed his life has an impact on the clinician. I have used the word, "fun," above. Sometimes it is that, but more often for me these conversations just give me a sense of awe, honor, and energy about the ways that people live their lives. As we have discussed, I believe that this effect is good for my own well-being and makes me a better clinician.

In being alert to people's competencies, we can give people credit for trying even if their efforts and accomplishments are off-base.

Clinician: *Made some dietary changes… cool…what have you done, in particular?*
Patient: *Well, the big thing in the last month is I switched from margarine to butter. I read that when the ingredients say "hydrolyzed" or "hydrolated" or whatever that is… it's not good. So I switched over to butter… organic butter, mind you… for all my cooking and rolls and muffins and toast and cookies…*
Clinician: *Wow, you read labels pretty carefully. Good for you for being so thoughtful about your nutrition. Can we talk a little about butter and maybe some other alternatives?*

Look for exceptions to problem states. A second approach to eliciting patients' wisdom about "how are you going to get there" is to explore exceptions to problem states… times when symptoms or problem patterns are *less* than other times.

A few words of background. The idea of the scientific and clinical value of exploring exceptions has its origins in the solution-focused therapy movement. Solution-focused therapy is an approach that grew out of the brief family therapy and problem-solving therapy movements of the 1970s. What began as a technique of "focused solution development" within the brief therapy context[2] evolved into an approach unto itself[3] and has prompted a lively literature in recent years.[4-8]

The fundamental scientific underpinning of solution-focused therapy, as I describe it to patients, students, and colleagues, is that no human experience remains constant in level or intensity over time. If you were to create a graph of the level or intensity of any experience on the Y axis, with "time" on the X axis, the graph would *never* be a flat line.

Your moods change over time… the graph is not a flat line. How many days per month (or week or year) you have a headache changes over time. Your ratings of satisfaction with your job changes over time. The number of minutes you spend flossing or brushing your teeth changes over time. No human experience is constant.

Changes in human experiences over time are not random; they happen for reasons. Perhaps you are late going to work, so you get in and out with the toothbrush. Perhaps your dentist has gently suggested that oral hygiene is not your strong suit, so you attend to dental care more thoroughly for a while. Perhaps you feel like you are really making a contribution in your workplace and your job satisfaction is high. Perhaps you have received no expressions of appreciation since your employer gave you the gift certificate for a free turkey last Thanksgiving and your job satisfaction is low.

If changes happen for reasons, then the conditions that prompt or promote meaningful changes are potentially reproducible.

The conversation in solution-focused approaches centers on re-producible changes. For a trivial human experience, such as cutting the grass, there will be times when you do the job more or less efficiently and when you are more or less satisfied with the result. You can think about what made the difference... height of cut, how much you overlapped rows, whether the mower was sharp, whether you just went back-and-forth or tried to make the pattern look like Fenway Park, and so forth... and reproduce approaches associated with greater efficiency or satisfaction.

For meaningful human experience, the conversation is the same.

- What makes the difference between times when your patient is hopeful about coping with cancer or not?
- When are the times when another patient has been more successful in managing his diabetes?
- If yet another patient with fibromyalgia could "fast forward" to a time when she was doing well with this, what would that look like?

Answers to such questions point to "solutions." What helps you sometimes to be more hopeful is a solution, as is what helps you to manage diabetes sometimes, as is what helps you to cope with fibromyalgia sometimes.

The emphasis in solution-focused conversations is on *exceptions* to problems. I am not particularly interested in when people are more depressed; I am interested in when they are less depressed. I am not as interested in when people have more headaches as I am in when they have fewer headaches, or perhaps handle them better. I am not interested in couples writing down details of their arguments with each other; I am interested in the times when they are a little more respectful, caring, and collaborative. I would focus less on why someone comes to the emergency room more frequently and more on what is going on over periods when they come to the emergency room less frequently.

By looking collaboratively at exceptions with patients, we honor and draw upon the wisdom from their life experiences.

My experience is that solution-focused conversations are clinically useful, affirming to patients, and certainly have a different energy compared with problem-focused conversations.

As a practical matter, exceptions can be pursued in the context of past experience or in the context of an envisioned future. The particular phrasing that I frequently use to explore past exceptions is *"when are the times when...?"*

- When have been the times when you have had fewer headaches?
- When were the times when your IBS was less troublesome?
- When have there been times when you have been less depressed and more confident?
- Tell me about some times when you have been... as you say, "more at one with the Universe."

There are two possible types of answers to such questions. Either patients will be able to describe the times when exceptions occurred and will be able to extract some meaningful ideas about why exceptions occurred, or they will be able to recall times when exceptions occurred but not be able to extract some meaningful ideas about why exceptions occurred.

If patients can identify times of exceptions and can extract ideas about how they brought these exceptions about, the conversation proceeds in the direction of *"go forth and do it again."*

Clinician: *So when has there been a time when you stopped smoking... do I recall that you stopped for two or three years at one point?*
Patient: *Good memory... actually it was about four years.*
Clinician: *How did you do it... how did you manage to be successful with that?*
Patient: *I was living in Pittsburgh, going to nursing school.*
Clinician: *Nursing school... usually that's a hard time for people.*
Patient: *Yea, it was hard, but it was really exciting to be learning all the things you learn in nursing school... that, and I had some really good friends in school with me.*

Clinician: *OK...*

Patient: *I think we were all pretty psyched up about being healthy, too... the instructors really emphasized that and we worked on it.*

Clinician: *Exciting to be learning things, good friends, support with other people for being healthy... are any of those things that you could be developing or re-connecting with at this point?*

If patients can identify times of exceptions and *can't* extract ideas about how they brought these exceptions about, the conversation proceeds in the direction of *"keep track and see what we can learn."*

Clinician: *Your idea of "feeling like my normal self..." when have been some times you can recall when you have felt a little more like your normal self?*

Patient: *Gee whiz, I don't know... it comes and goes.*

Clinician: *When was the last time you remember that you felt a little more like your normal self?*

Patient: *Um... probably some time last week.*

Clinician: *Do you recall any particular day or circumstance?*

Patient: *Nothing stands out.*

Clinician: *OK, fair enough. I understand that how much you feel like yourself varies a lot day to day, right?*

Patient: *Right.*

Clinician: *Let me suggest that you keep track for a couple of weeks and see what we can learn from that. Would you be up for that?*

Patient: *OK.*

Clinician: *All right... let me suggest that you write down every night how much you felt like yourself each day... you can make up your own scale or words. The write down any thoughts you have about why you may have felt like that on each day and maybe a couple of things that you did that you wonder whether they may have been important...*

Exceptions can also be pursued in the context of an envisioned future:

Clinician: *OK, let's think about this goal of "accepting your health." You can't do as much as you used to but you want to figure out how to accept your health and your health limitations as they are, right?*
Patient: *Yea... I used to be into judo, running... I can't do that stuff any more.*
Clinician: *OK. Let me ask you this... picture yourself in the future... maybe a few months from now... still not able to do judo or running or things like that, but accepting your health 50% more than you do now. What does that look like?*
Patient: *I'm more peaceful... a lot more peaceful... not as angry...*
Clinician: *And what are you doing, now that you are more peaceful?*
Patient: *I'd be reading to my kids more... I'd probably have chilled enough that I could really spend some time with them.*
Clinician: *Good, really connecting with your kids...*

The envisioned future points to some possible exceptions to the anger and non-acceptance that this patient has been feeling. The clinician's premise... which is probably accurate... is that this patient's meaningfully connecting with her kids will probably help her acceptance of her health and health limitations.

This underscores, by the way, the relationship of mutual influence between feelings and behavior. Most of us naturally relate to the idea that feelings influence behavior, and also to the reciprocal idea that behavior influences feelings. Being depressed or being energetic might influence whether we would visit with friends, and whether we visit with friends might influence whether we feel depressed or energetic. For purposes of identifying exceptions to problem states and potential directions for "how do you get there," the sequence is:

1. If you felt better, what would you do?
2. Do what you would do if you felt better.
3. Increase the likelihood of feeling better.

Use scaling. A third approach to eliciting patients' wisdom about "how are you going to get there" is making use of self-appraisal scales as reference points to explore lessons learned from variations in patients' experiences over time.

The core question, as I typically phrase it, is:

> *Think of a scale of zero to ten, with zero standing for "the pits" and ten not standing for "perfect and wonderful," but "I feel pretty good about how I'm doing... life has its ups and downs, but I'm generally going in a good direction." With respect to the goals we have talked about, where would you put yourself on that scale today?*

I use the awkward language for "ten," by the way, because I prefer to have the top of the scale not stand for "perfection," and therefore to be attainable. This is a completely subjective scale, but it is fascinating to me that the number that crosses my mind as I ask patients this question is almost never more than one unit away from what they say, and more often than not hits it on the nose.

Having this numerical self-appraisal, clinicians can explore behavioral and attitudinal correlates of patients' ratings and variations over time.

Clinician: *Think of a scale of zero to ten, with zero standing for "the pits" and ten not standing for "perfect and wonderful," but "I feel pretty good about how I'm doing... life has its ups and downs, but I'm generally going in a good direction." With respect to how you see yourself coping with your grandmother's death, where would you put yourself on that scale today?*
Patient: *Six.*
Clinician: *OK... and when you called to set up this appointment at the end of last week, where would you have put yourself on the scale?*
Patient: *Oh, man... three... two.*
Clinician: *So... you gained three to four points between the time you called to set up this visit and today?*
Patient: *Yea, I guess...*
Clinician: *Cool. So what did you do in the last six or seven days to get yourself another three or four points on the scale?*

Patient: *I was really freaked out last week… with my parents both in the bag most of the time… my grandmother was really the one that raised me… the one I turned to…*

Clinician: *Yea, I know how much she meant to you. But let's look at how you've moved up on the scale since then… what was it that you did that helped you to move forward like that?*

Patient: *Well, I have some good friends who keep telling me it's going to be OK. But to be honest, I think the turning point was going to the cemetery this weekend and just talking to her. I know it sounds stupid, but I really had the sense that she was there telling me that I'm ready to live my life.*

Clinician: *Wow… doesn't sound stupid at all. And when you think about being "ready to live your life," what does that mean to you?*

Here, the clinician elicits the patient's self-appraisal that he has moved forward with the goal of coping with his grandmother's death and invites the patient to say more about what "ready to live my life" means. The clinician's intent is to turn the conversation… and the patient's attention… to attitudes, behaviors and values that would comprise living life meaningfully. More good spiritual care… helping patients to connect to things that matter to them.

The additional way that I find scaling particularly useful with the "how are you going to get there" question is in the exploration of gradual or sequential future changes. A minute later into the conversation with the patient whose grandmother died:

Clinician: *So you're at a "six" today. Good. I respect what you're saying about how you have been courageous in facing this in the last few days. Let me ask you… if you were at a "seven" instead of a "six," what would that look like? How would that be different from a "six?"*

Patient: *Oh, I can tell you that… the next thing I need to do is to start to go through her stuff. My folks won't do it and I really don't want them to. Pictures, books… all those things… going through her clothes and giving them away. It's not going to be easy, but I have to do it and maybe I'm getting to the point where I can.*

The behavioral correlate of "seven," processing the grandmother's effects, will be both a measure of continued progress and a specific task or methodology to cultivate that progress.

Scaling questions about past and future variations can be used in countless ways:

- *Where were you on the scale at your complete low point? What did that look like?*
- *What is the highest you have been on the scale in the last year? What were you like at that point?*
- *When you are at an "eight" instead of a "three" or "four," what in particular is different about your attitude... how do you tend to see things differently at those times?*
- *Where would you hope to be in six months with your goal of "figuring out who Michelle is?" What would you be seeing in yourself... your attitudes and what you are doing... that would tell you that you're there?*

Just ask... theory and sense. The fourth approach to eliciting patients' wisdom about "how are you going to get there" is just to ask directly for this wisdom.

- *What is your theory about what is going on with these emotional times and what you'll need to be doing to move through them?*
- *What is your sense about how you're going to keep going being an encourager and supporter in your crazy workplace?*

A physician assistant recounts:

I saw a woman, late twenties, three months postpartum, who came in having had a serious panic attack. She was going to work... she did telephone sales for our local internet service provider... when she developed sweats, dizziness, difficulty breathing. She called a friend who brought her to the ER, where they did some cardiac screening and concluded that she had had a panic attack. They gave her some benzos and told her to follow up here. I just asked her what she thought was going on and if she had any ideas about what could help her get a little more settled. She said that she had thought about that and wondered if this episode was telling her that she should be staying home with her child. As we talked about it, it sounded pretty clear-cut apart from the income issue. First child... she had always wanted to be a mom and it was devastating to leave her daughter every morning. There was no love lost for her work, either... she felt like she was always under the gun to make sales and always had somebody looking over her shoulder. I thought that made a lot of sense. She and her husband talked it over and decided they could make a go of it on his income, so she quit her job and did really well.

Questions about patients' "theories" or "sense" of what is going on and how they can be approaching the circumstances they face are generally low-cost and high-gain. If patients *don't* have particular theories about what's going on and how they are going to move in directions that are important to them, you're not far behind for having asked. If patients *do* have some theories or sense about how they can be getting where they want to go, however, it can help clinicians to get to the heart of the matter in an efficient way.

STRATEGY 14
Elicit patients' wisdom and competence

Invite patients to talk about what they have learned from their own life experience, particularly the more successful times... and their ideas about how they can best be proceeding with the things that matter to them.

Wisdom from clinicians

Recall again the template for spiritual care conversations:

1. Where do you want to go?
2. How are you going to get there?
   a. wisdom from patients
   b. wisdom from clinicians

3. What are the next steps?

We look, now, at "2b."

Patients, appropriately, look to clinicians for wisdom and expertise. When I fell down our icy steps last winter and injured my shoulder… I wish it had been a more glorious athletically-related injury, but that's the way it goes in Maine in January… I consulted my colleague and friend down the hall who is boarded in Sports Medicine. I was not looking for him to elicit my wisdom about the diagnosis and healing; I was looking to him to tell me what was wrong and prescribe a plan for treatment and rehabilitation.

In the health care world, we often use the rubric of "patient education" to describe the communication of our own expertise and wisdom to patients. We "educate" patients about self-care, management of acute and chronic illnesses, expectations about surgery and rehabilitation, and so forth.

It always seems to me that the phrase "patient education" needs a context. What clinicians do in communicating their own wisdom to patients is more than just providing information; it is searching for or developing *ways* of communicating our wisdom that people can hear.

There are three ways of expressing this wisdom that I find useful.

This is what the data say. The approach that is probably deeply ingrained for most of us as clinicians is to express our wisdom to patients in the form of data. There are data about nutritional recommendations for cardiac disease. There are data about behavioral, pharmacological, and integrative treatments for depression. There are data about osteopathic manipulation for various types of somatic dysfunction.

When patients come to us with meaningful life and health goals, part of our response to the question of "how are you going to get there" is to report results or summaries of research. We can report data in dispassionate, objective terms or with more pizzazz.

The dispassionate approach:

As I review the research about people coping with chronic pain, the three recurrent themes I see are relaxation, activity scheduling and problem-solving. Let me say a few words about each of these and we can talk about where you think you might wish to go from here...

The more-pizzazz approach:

We're talking about the idea that pain is not "in your head," but that things in your life do affect your experience of pain. There's a cool example of this in research from World War II that I like to describe to patients. Researchers identified a large group of soldiers who had had battlefield injuries that were serious but not fatal... people who had lost arms or legs, who had serious head wounds, and so forth. For this group of people, they searched out a comparable number of stateside civilians who had comparable injuries... people who had lost arms or legs or sustained serious head wounds in motor vehicle accidents, for instance. Then they asked these groups of people for their self-ratings of pain. For the same injuries... battlefield versus stateside... what they found is that the soldiers reported significantly less pain than the civilians. There was no physiological reason for them to experience less pain, since the injuries were the same. The researchers' conclusion was that the difference was what the injuries meant to these two groups of people. If you are a comfortable civilian and you lose an arm in a motor vehicle accident, your world is turned upside down and what you see is disability stretching out in front of you. If you are a soldier and lose an arm in combat, this means that you are going to get a medical discharge, survive the war, and get a ticket home to people you love... probably a pretty good tradeoff for most people in Sicily or Normandy or Guadalcanal.

I say "pizzazz;" this type of approach to reporting data emphasizes the human context and significance and, as in the example of the matched control pain research, engages the listener with a narrative.

This is what my patients have said. Patients are often captivated and moved by the experience of other patients. As with the reporting of data, clinicians can communicate the experience of other patients in more global and summary form, or in more personal, narrative form.

The global/summary approach:

As I talk with couples about the kinds of restoration of their relationships that the two of you are considering, I look for what makes the difference between couples that make it and couples that don't. One of the consistent things I notice over the years is that the couples that don't make it put a lot of effort into trying to change the other person. The couples that make it put their effort into exploring how they can change to become better partners.

The more personal, narrative form:

I had a patient a while ago who had been raped. She thought she knew the person well enough to be safe with him, but she was wrong. It was one of those cases where she didn't report the rape soon enough to gather the appropriate evidence to make a viable legal case, so the man was never prosecuted. He immediately dropped out of her life and she didn't have any contact with him or feel in any danger, but she struggled with being furious with him. She felt rage for weeks and weeks after the event and found herself ruminating about all sorts of ways she could extract revenge. Being a peaceful sort, she knew she wouldn't act on these thoughts of revenge, but they haunted her… kept her up at night. She saw her friends less and less and started missing work. This went on for several months. Then she said that one night she heard a voice saying to her, "The best revenge is living a good life." She didn't know quite what to make of this, but she thought about it for a couple of days and says that it dawned on her that the more she pulled back in living her life and allowed herself to be preoccupied with the rape, the more she kept the rapist in the position of violating her. By "living a good life," she took away his power over her.

Like the narrative description of the matched control pain study, stories about patients can captivate the attention of listeners. For most listeners, there would be a qualitative difference between a clinician expressing the concept *"It's important to go on living your life and not give him power over you"* and the clinician expressing the same wisdom in the form of the narrative.

Narratives, of course, have to safeguard patients' confidentiality. There are a few patients over the years who have specifically invited me to tell their stories, even with personal identification, but I routinely disguise the particulars of stories in such a way that real people are not recognizable.

This is what I have learned from my experience. We are clinicians, and we are also human beings. The fact that you are reading this sentence, having picked up this book, suggests to me that self-reflection and self-awareness are values that are important to you. If this is the case, then the observations and insights from your own life may comprise part of the bank of wisdom from which you share ideas with patients.

Much of what I suggest to people about mindfulness, for instance, arises as much out of my personal life experience as it does out of reading or clinical experience. The idea of focusing mindful attention, without judgment, on this present moment has served me well with all of the concerns, questions, and doubts that all of us a human beings face.

Similarly, I have found that for myself, strategies of distraction from distress work less well than strategies of mindful engagement with something that matters to me. If I am personally preoccupied with something, I can distract myself by listening to a couple of innings of the Red Sox on the radio, but the preoccupation is still there when I turn the radio off. (And, of course, if it turns out that the Sox are getting blown out, listening to the game introduces another layer of problems that severely tax my ability to be mindful.)

Instead of temporary distraction, however, I find that mindful engagement with something that matters to me... caring about my wife, calling my children, being a good neighbor, writing some paragraphs of a book... has a much more profound impact on my preoccupations.

It is fair game and it is meaningful to express this kind of wisdom from our own experience in spiritual care conversations as long as doing so serves the health and well-being of the patient. In a context where the conversation continues to be *about the patient*, our disclosure of our own experiences and wisdom can be compelling for patients and can help us as clinicians to come across in a more genuine way. If the context switches and the conversation becomes *about us*, it ceases to be therapeutic for the patient and it is important to return the focus to the patient's hopes and goals.

STRATEGY 15
Express your own wisdom in some new ways

In addition to customary approaches to "patient education," experiment with expressing your wisdom in narrative forms and in sharing some lessons from your own life experience.

NEXT STEPS

The first element in spiritual care conversations has to do with defining with patients where they wish to be going. The second element has to do with defining how they are going to get there. The final element has to do with inviting patients to make commitments about next steps.

Conversation about next steps in spiritual care is important for two reasons. First, *this is how change happens*. Change... or, more broadly, people making choices that arise out of values, goals and approaches that are important to them... happens away from health care encounters. Any of us can have compassionate and brilliant spiritual care conversations with patients, but unless patients somehow follow up on these conversations in their lives away from us, not much will happen.

The second reason is that *change is generative.* Change begets further change. Small changes create energy, optimism and momentum, which often translate into more substantial changes. A retired man, for instance, had experienced a painful divorce after many years of being together with his wife. He believed that he needed to "make a new life" for himself as a single person, but found that it was very hard to get going on some of the ideas he had about how he could be approaching this. He did not much go out, although he believed this would be beneficial. He did not cultivate some of the friendships that had survived the divorce, although he believed this would be beneficial as well. He did not put much effort into keeping up his house, as he and his wife had always done. The turning point for this man came when he decided to do his dishes. All of the two or three sets of dinnerware and utensils that he owned had been stacked up, unattended, beside the sink. One morning, he said, he decided that he had had enough and that it was time to go to work. He spent the morning cleaning it all up and commented, "It sounds silly to talk about dishes, but doing that convinced me that maybe I really could get on with making a different life." Which he subsequently did.

Approaches to next steps. Let me suggest three approaches to the process of pursuing next steps that I have found useful in spiritual care conversations.

Jot down reactions. The least demanding option in terms of defining next steps is to invite people to think about the conversations that they have had. My experience is that the additional step of asking patients to "jot down" reactions adds an element of accountability and usually results in some more substantive reflection on conversations than there is with the simpler invitation to "think about it."

You've both said that you're a little concerned about what kinds of parent you will be after your child arrives. The fact that you're asking this question... and what I know from seeing you together... make me think that you'll do fine. But let's look at this just a little more. Between now and your next OB visit, let me invite you to think about how you'd put into words what you would like to be like as parents... and jot down some ideas and bring them along.

Keep track. Particularly when clinicians and patients wish to understand something better, or when there is no readily apparent strategy to pursue for patients to move forward with goals that are meaningful for them, we can ask patients to keep track of the way things happen.

I appreciate what you're saying about finding more "dignity" in how you deal with your pain. We're kicking around some ideas about what that might look like, but at this point, it would be helpful for me to see how this plays out in the next couple of weeks to understand it better. Before your next clinic visit on the 26th, I'd like you to spend a couple of minutes every night, looking back on the day and writing a few notes about anything you did that represents some degree of dignity for you. Let's see what you notice and see what we can learn together.

Asking patients to keep track often results in clinically useful information. Beyond that, this assignment will sometimes become a useful intervention, because keeping track of some valued events tends to result in increases in those events. Asking a patient to keep track of his spending quality time with his child, for instance, will typically result in more quality time... because this is important enough to the patient to be talking about it and because he is specifically paying attention to this.

Do something different. The core feature of approaches to next steps is, simply, to do something different. I'm not sure it even always matters *what* people do differently, so much as *that* they change something about the patterns in their lives, building on what matters to them. Changing something specific about how one relates to a partner or child. Changing something specific about how one spends time. Making a concrete change in what one eats.

As I have suggested, doing something different generates energy and optimism; when you see something change as a result of your discretionary action, it feels hopeful. Doing something different also adds a feedback loop to the whole process of spiritual care conversations that we have been considering because it gathers wisdom and direction. When you start moving, you often get a clearer picture of where you are, where you want to go, and how you're going to get there.

We've talked about a number of issues in your life that your illness has prompted you to pursue at this point... your relationship with your mom, backing off at work, getting back into some of the creative pursuits that have been important for you before... among these things, what would you see yourself particularly putting some energy into in the next three or four weeks?

There may be an answer to this question in the conversation; there may not. If the patient has some sense of what he or she could be doing to follow up on the conversation, then this becomes the next step.

I think that the idea of your doing [whatever it is] is great and I want to support you experimenting with this between now and when we next get together.

If the patient does not have a clear sense of this, the next step can be to decide on a specific item of follow up.

In the next day or so, I'd like you to decide for yourself about one or two specific things you want to do to follow up on this conversation. I'll look forward to hearing.

My practice is that I fairly consistently write down for patients our collaborative agreement about next steps. I use a quarter sheet of letter-sized paper and write a few words about wisdom (from the patient and from me, as we have discussed) and next steps. Example:

- *Talking it out, rather than shutting down*
- *Facing things, rather than pushing them away*
- *Choose some follow-up about*
  - *exercise*
  - *calming practices*

The first two items reflect the patient's language for principles that she wishes to be cultivating in her life. The third item reflects our collaborative agreement that she will choose and pursue some specific follow-up of our conversation about exercise and various calming practices.

Back in the days when we had paper records, I had quarter-sheet paper made up in NCR (no carbon required) format; I would give the patient the original copy of the summary notes and tape the yellow NCR copy in the record. Now that we are in the electronic medical record era, I give the copy of the summary note to the patient and type (or dictate) the summary from the yellow copy into the electronic record.

STRATEGY 16
Collaborate with patients in defining next steps

Invite patients' wisdom and decisions about how they could best put energy into following up with the goals and approaches from their conversations with you.

SUMMARY

A template for spiritual care conversations;

- Goals: What matters to you and where do you want to go?
  - Outcomes or values
  - Rooted in the "vital and sacred"
  - Within patients' control

- o Positively framed
- o Using patients' language
- o Directed toward three choices
  - Change the circumstances
  - Cope with the circumstances
  - Be healthy and whole in spite of whatever is going on with distressing circumstances
- o Moving patients beyond complaints
- Approaches: How are you going to get there?
  - o Wisdom from patients
    - Catch patients in the act of being competent
    - Look for exceptions to problem states
    - Use scaling
    - Just ask; theory and sense
  - o Wisdom from clinicians
    - This is what the data say
    - This is what my patients have said
    - This is what I have learned from my experience
- Next steps
  - o Jot down reactions
  - o Keep track
  - o Do something different

REFERENCES

1. Wheatley M. *Turning to One Another: Simple Conversations to Restore Hope to the Future.* San Francisco: Berrett-Koehler; 2002.

2. De Shazer S, Berg I, Lipchick E, et al. Brief therapy: Focused solution development. *Fam Process.* 1986;25(207-21).

3. Molnar A, De Shazer S. Solution-focused therapy: Toward the identification of therapeutic tasks. *J Mar Fam Ther.* 1987;13(4):349-358.

4. Walter J, Peller J. *Becoming Solution-focused in Brief Therapy.* New York: Brunner/Mazel; 1992.

5. O'Hanlon W, Weiner-Davis M. *In Search of Solutions: A New Direction in Psychotherapy.* New York: W. W. Norton; 1989.

6. Friedman S. *The New Language of Change.* New York: Guilford;

1993.

7. Duncan B, Hubble M, Miller S. *Psychotherapy with "Impossible" Cases: The Efficient Treatment of Therapy Veterans.* New York: W. W. Norton; 1997.

8. Walter J, Peller J. *Recreating Brief Therapy.* New York: W. W. Norton; 2000.

Chapter Ten

Be Attuned to Recurring Themes of Transcendence and Valued Directions

All the greatest and most important problems of life are fundamentally insoluble. They can never be solved, but only outgrown. This "outgrowing" proves on further investigation to require a new level of consciousness. Some higher or wider interest appeared on the horizon and through this broadening of outlook the insoluble problem lost its urgency. It was not solved logically in its own terms but faded when confronted with a new and stronger life urge.

Carl Jung

In outward appearance, Joanne looked like any other nursing student, although a few years older than most of her peers. Her personal journey had been more distinctive. Growing up in a home where both of her parents had been emotionally and often physically absent, she largely fended for herself since her childhood years. She had been sexually abused from ages 10 to 12 by an uncle who eventually was hauled off to prison for armed robbery. Struggling with substance abuse, Joanne had been driving drunk when she was 17 when she lost control of her car on an icy road, flipping the car several times, resulting in the death of her best friend, who was her passenger. As a young adult, she suffered from lupus and from periodic flashbacks to the abuse and the accident. Now in her late twenties, she had an on and off relationship with a boyfriend, but clearly the passionate urge in her life was to become a nurse. "I decided," she said, "that I couldn't bring my friend back or change any of what's happened or make my lupus go away, but I could make my life count from here on."

For all of us as human beings, much of life experience is beyond our control. Only rarely do we relate to life with the degree of certainty associated with fixing a leaky faucet or sawing a board in half. As situations involve other people or the natural world... or even some emotional and cognitive processes within ourselves... our ability to control what happens with any degree of certainty becomes tenuous.

In Joanne's case, there were powerful *external events*... absent parents and sexual abuse by an uncle... that were assuredly beyond her control. She also faced cognitive and emotional *internal events*... flashbacks about trauma, feelings of sadness or guilt about bad choices... that tend to be fairly persistent for most people. And she wrestled with *physiological* experiences associated with lupus where she had some modest success attenuating symptoms such as fatigue, inflammation, and rash, while dealing with the reality, as she said, that the disease itself was probably not going to go away.

The premise that much of life experience is not controllable goes down hard. I sometimes wonder if we have a collective sense of psychological manifest destiny. Patients that I see frequently come to me wishing to somehow change experiences that are not very changeable. The distressed woman who wishes to change her husband. The disabled drywall installer who wishes to have his lower back pain go away. The office worker who exists in an extraordinarily stressful environment who wishes to rid himself of the relentless worries that keep him up at night.

The problem, as we discussed in Chapter 9, is that efforts to change the circumstances that come at us often do not work. More than that, efforts to change external and internal circumstances can be counterproductive. The more people try not to be anxious, the more anxious they become. An approach of I'M NOT GOING TO BE ANXIOUS... NOW I'M GOING TO RELAX creates anxiety more often than it calms it.

Same thing interpersonally. I'm a nice guy, but frankly, the more you try to change me into your image of what I should be, the more set in my own ways I am likely to become.

A patient who is active in 12-step programs, in fact, recently gave me a new addition to my collection of AA aphorisms; "what you resist persists." The more you try to change unchangeable things, the more they push back at you. Good wisdom.

The alternative, according to Joanne, is to somehow let go or make peace with that which is not changeable, and to move on with current life choices in a meaningful way. As she says, she can't change her history or make her lupus go away, but she can "make my life count from here on."

TRANSCENDENCE AND VALUED DIRECTIONS

Joanne's journey and commitment point to recurrent themes in spiritual care; transcendence and valued directions. Spiritual care often encourages people with *transcendence*... the journey of letting go or making peace with the unchangeable elements of life. And spiritual care encourages people to be moving in *valued directions*... making meaningful life choices and finding meaningful life paths.

Our modern word "transcendence" originates in the Latin "transcendere;" to climb, step, or go across or over. These spatial images suggest three key elements of transcendence.

First, *transcendence does not mean avoidance of pain and suffering; it means facing pain and suffering.* When you "go across or over," you are not staying at home and you are not choosing an alternate route. Driving east to Maine after my last sabbatical at the Program in Integrative Medicine at the University of Arizona School of

Medicine, my wife and I made the arduous journey over thirty miles of washboard unpaved roads to Chaco Culture National Historical Park. Chaco was a major center of ancestral Puebloan culture in northwestern New Mexico, flourishing for about three hundred years beginning in the mid-800s. It remains... probably thanks to its remoteness... an extraordinarily well preserved example of ancient American building and community life. To this day, you can hold a two-foot level up against the masonry border of a window opening that was laid a thousand years ago and not see much of the light of day.

Chaco is thought to have been at the hub of an extended network of communications and trading around the region. As a matter of scientific and probably religious purity, the Chacoan engineers charted directions to other centers such as Mesa Verde and created routes between centers that were absolutely straight. No curves, no switchbacks, no detours... straight. If the route encountered a cliff face, so be it; the ancient road builders created steps or handholds. "Transcendence," for the Chacoans, literally meant "going over" and resisting the temptation to choose an alternate route.

Second, *transcendence does not mean distraction from pain and suffering; it means looking it full in the face and thereby robbing it of its power.* A patient recounts,

> *I always had the image that there were these terrible dark forces inside of me... things that were planted there from my years of abuse... and whenever I would get some sense of them forcing their way to the surface, I would furiously get busy doing something... cleaning, cooking, cutting the grass... to keep from facing them because I thought it would be too terrible. Then I guess I got to the point where I was just putting too much energy into not facing these things, so I began to say "Go ahead, come on." I remember one day just being flooded with the image of my husband beating me and I just let it come and be there... and it was amazing that the more I stayed with it and let it be there, the more its power went away. This was really the turning point for me*

when I realized that keeping myself protected from my fears just made them bigger, and facing my fears made them smaller.

This proposition... that facing suffering and having it be what it is takes away its power... reflects spiritual wisdom from across the centuries. In the Christian tradition, for instance, sixteenth century Spanish mystic John of the Cross wrote about embracing and moving through the "Dark Night of the Soul" as part of a journey toward ultimate transformation and union with God.

Third, *transcendence does not mean coming to a stop*. The verbs "to climb, step, or go across or over" all entail continuing motion and forward movement. There may be *pausing* associated with transcendence... you pause to meditate, reflect, or to gather courage... but you do not stop. Joanne did not stop with the recognition that she couldn't change her past or her illness; she directed her passion and energy toward making her life count in a prospective career in nursing.

Pursuing valued directions, therefore, is a vitally important part of the spiritual process of relating to life circumstances outside of our control.

Transcendence and the pursuit of valued directions go together. They are complementary. We "go across or over" and we move toward something that matters. We let go of the binding energy of uncontrollable pain and suffering, and we move, as Jung says, in the direction of a "new and stronger life urge."

SPIRITUAL CARE TOWARD TRANSCENDENCE AND VALUED DIRECTIONS

OK. Let's get back to clinical reality. I have a Maine friend and colleague, Kenneth H. Hamilton, MD, who is a former surgeon who has for many years developed programs of peer support for people with a variety of medical and personal struggles.[1,2] He poses the core question, "Life is giving you this challenge... now, where would you like to go with your life?"

A great clinical question... a spiritual question... for all sorts of human struggles that we see:

- The 40 year old bank manager with a new diagnosis of ALS
- The 23 year old mother of two who is subject to domestic violence
- The 60 year old woman, a year post-stroke, who struggles with the suffering of not being her "normal self" and not knowing whether this will ever return.
- The 28 year old former Marine who suffered several episodes of concussive trauma from bomb blasts in Iraq who finds himself unable to concentrate in a sufficiently sustained way to work.

What does it mean to provide good spiritual care to these people? How do we help and support them to somehow transcend the parts of their lives that are beyond their control and to move in directions of meaning and purpose?

For the rest of this chapter, I want to explore some specific pathways to transcendence and to pursuing valued directions. Let's look at some of the particulars, then I want to suggest at the end of the chapter how this fits in with the issues and approaches we have considered so far.

APPROACHES TO TRANSCENDENCE

A variety of approaches to transcendence are presented in the sidebar. There is substantial overlap among these approaches, but they differ linguistically, and some will resonate more than others with individual patients.

Approaches to transcendence

- Letting go
- Willingness/acceptance
- Mindfulness/being present
- Non-attachment
- Serenity
- Spiritual surrender
- Gratitude/gratefulness
- Forgiveness

Letting go

I list this first because letting go seems to be the most prominent among these approaches in the popular consciousness. Google, for instance, provides 19,400,000 hits (in 0.15 seconds, I might add). I also frequently hear the language and rubric of letting go from patients, particularly in the context of painful emotions and past suffering.

Patient: *I just can't believe it… we were married for 11 years and it felt like things were pretty good to me, then she just came to me one day and said she wanted out. I don't know… maybe we were drifting apart, but the things she said to me about how I was failing her all the time really hurt. So now, here we are, haggling over who gets the house and who gets the dog.*
Clinician: *Wow, a real shock to you… so what do you do now?*
Patient: *I just do it all through my lawyer… I told him to tell her she can have the house… I wouldn't want to stay in the house anyway… but I do want the dog. She's probably my best friend.*
Clinician: *Yea, pursuing those things… OK… what do you do about the shock and the hurt of all of this crashing down so suddenly… out of the blue?*
Patient: *Let it go.*

Clinician: *Let it go... what does that mean to you?*
Patient: *She's not going to change at this point and I can either let it drag me down or I can get on with my life.*
Clinician: *Drag you down... so if you don't let it go, what is that like?*
Patient: *I don't know how to stop being angry, but I know I can't live there because it's eating me up.*
Clinician: *It does you in to dwell on how you feel she's treated you.*
Patient: *Yea, and it doesn't get me anywhere.*
Clinician: *OK... you talk about "getting on with your life" and "getting somewhere..." say more about what this means to you...*

The clinician here picks up on the patient's reference to "letting go" and explores what this means. The answer has two key elements.

First, the patient says that *not* letting go has a substantial personal cost. Dwelling on how his wife treated him would "eat him up."

I find that exploring the cost of being stuck on challenging life events... in this case, the cost of not letting go... is often a fruitful foundation in conversations about transcendence.

Clinician: *Being, as you say, "preoccupied" with how your boss passed over you... how is that for you?*
Patient: *It's terrible... keeps me up at night, keeps me from really focusing on the stuff I need to do...*
Clinician: *I understand something about what it's like for you to go through this, but it sounds like it's not helping to be preoccupied with it... is that right?*
Patient: *Absolutely.*

Second, the conversation about letting go with the patient whose wife left him turns to his ideas of "getting on with life" and "getting somewhere." He is not sure, at this point, how he will stop being angry, but he is aware that moving forward will be part of the solution. My experience is that the *valued directions part of the package...* like Jung's idea of the "new and stronger life urge..." often helps with the *transcendence part of the package.* For this particular patient, part of "getting on with life" for this eventually involved leadership in a support program for single people, and the passionate and committed involvement that he brought to this program was significantly healing for him.

CLINICAL TIPS: Much of my conversations with people about "letting go" follows the approaches to "where do you want to go" and eliciting patients' wisdom about "how are you going to get there" from Chapter 9.

- *When you say "letting go," what does that mean to you?*
- *As you are able to let go a little more, how do you picture being different?*
- *When have been the times when you have let go to some extent and how have you done that?*
- *What is your sense about the main thing you will need to be doing to move more toward letting go at this point?*

Willingness/acceptance

Like "letting go," "acceptance" is part of the common language of personal experience:

"I need to accept the fact that I have diabetes and make the best of it."

"Willingness," in contrast, is a more specific word that arises largely out of the literature on Acceptance and Commitment Therapy (ACT).[3, 4] ACT theorists and practitioners refer to themselves as "third generation behavior therapists," the first generation being rats in Skinner boxes... the focus on learning theory and observable behavior... and the second generation bringing the incorporation of cognitive events and cognitive change... such as the "Rational-emotive Therapy" of Albert Ellis and the "Cognitive Therapy" of Aaron Beck.

The third generation clearly changes course. Rather than focusing on changing observable behavior or private cognitions and assumptions, ACT focuses on acceptance of uncontrollable and unwanted events ("acceptance"), and on living with purpose and dignity in the presence of uncontrollable and unwanted events ("commitment").

The literature about ACT particularly addresses internal and subjective events such as anxiety,[5] worry,[6] and pain.[7] The premise is that it is precisely the attempt to control such internal events that a) doesn't work, b) causes distress, and c) robs people of the opportunity to live meaningfully. You have probably seen, as have I many times, for instance, people who struggle with anxiety and whose attempts to control anxiety leave them lonely and bored inside homes where they feel safe.

"Willingness," in this context, means working with people to abandon the quest for controlling uncontrollable and unwanted thoughts, feelings and somatic experiences, to be "willing" to have their experience be what it is, and to devote their energy toward living in ways that matter to them.

A patient from last week:

I have aching in my joints, pain in my back… it's been that way for years and years and I don't see it changing. I've learned that I just can't fight it anymore… it's going to be there and I can't spend my life wishing it wasn't. So I've got to do the best I can… hang out with friends, do some singing, do some writing… pace myself.

For this person, giving up the quest to control pain and make it go away frees her to follow social and creative pursuits.

ACT in practice is a spirited enterprise, with a great deal of action, specialized exercises, metaphors and humor. For those of us who are not ACT therapists, the moral of the story is that giving up the quest to control unwanted thoughts, feelings, and somatic experiences… being willing to experience them as they are… frees people like the woman with chronic pain to devote more energy to meaningful living.

CLINICAL TIPS: My suggestion is that pursuing a "willingness" approach to transcendence in spiritual care conversations can include three practical elements.

First, it can be practical and helpful to invite patients to consider the possibility that attempting to control the uncontrollable doesn't work and doesn't help.

Clinician: *So you've struggled with this pain for a long time.*
Patient: *Sure have. It stays there and stays there… it's always there… it's really wearing me down.*
Clinician: *What sorts of things have you done to try to get rid of it?*
Patient: *I usually try to distract myself with something… watch TV, do video games…*
Clinician: *How does that work?*
Patient: *Maybe I'll get into some TV show, but lots of times the pain's still there and it's always back when the show is over.*
Clinician: *You distract yourself, but it doesn't make any lasting difference?*
Patient: *Yea.*
Clinician: *What else have you tried?*
Patient: *Lying down, hot soaks… maybe the soaks help a little… I took Oxycodone for a couple of years and that helped some.*
Clinician: *What happened with the Oxycodone?*
Patient: *I came up with pot in my urine and that violated my narcotic contract, so my last doctor stopped prescribing it for me.*
Clinician: *OK. So it sounds like the best I'm hearing in your experience is "helps some." At this point, do you think it's possible that your pain may go away?*
Patient: *Sure hasn't shown any signs of it.*
Clinician: *So do you see it as something that you'll have to figure out a way to live with?*

Patient: *I guess so… that's what I've been doing.*
Clinician: *OK. Let's talk about what your experience has been with the times when you have been able to live with it a little better…*

This is the conversation about "doesn't work." The clinician establishes the fact that the patient has made a variety of efforts that all fall short of the patient's hope that the pain would go away. Clinicians can also have a conversation about "doesn't help."

Clinician: *How do you deal with the anxiety episodes that you're describing?*
Patient: *Mainly I try to make them not happen.*
Clinician: *And how do you do that?*
Patient: *I mostly stay at home.*
Clinician: *Stay at home?*
Patient: *Yea, I feel safe there.*
Clinician: *What do you do… how do you pass the time?*
Patient: *Oh, I don't know… I do my housework, watch TV.*
Clinician: *How is that for you?*
Patient: *OK I guess… it's what I do.*
Clinician: *You don't sound particularly enthusiastic.*
Patient: *Would you be enthusiastic about staying home and watching TV?*
Clinician: *It's not very inspiring for you… OK… so staying protected from anxiety leads you to this life at home that you feel pretty uninspired about… how would you be spending your time if you were not limited by anxiety?*
Patient: *Working, I guess… out in the world.*
Clinician: *And what difference would that make to you?*
Patient: *I'd at least be accomplishing something.*
Clinician: *I want to understand what you mean by that, but first… let me check out what I'm hearing… keeping yourself protected from anxiety leads you to have a more restricted and uninspiring life than you would hope to have, is that right?*

Here the clinician takes up the point that the patient's quest for control of anxiety keeps his life small. The clinician is headed toward exploring with the patient what he means by "accomplishing something," to open up future possibilities that could be available if the patient were to pursue a path of willingness.

The second practical element of a "willingness" approach to transcendence in spiritual care conversations is to provide some perspective on the idea that suspending the quest to control unwanted experiences and facing them takes away their power. Sometimes patients will have life experiences that demonstrate this.

Clinician: *Has there been a time for you when you remember having been willing to take on some uncomfortable feelings in order to do what you needed or really wanted to do?*

Patient: *Hm. You know, what comes to mind is running for student council in eighth grade. I really wanted to be on student council, but it required me to give a speech in front of the whole school. I was really freaked out, but somehow I did it.*

Clinician: *How did that feel?*

Patient: *Wow, I haven't thought about that for years. I remember... it felt really great.*

Clinician: *How would you put into words what you learned from that?*

Other times, the conversation may grow out of our own life experience, as I suggested in the last chapter. A story I tell frequently:

One semester in graduate school, I signed on to be a teaching assistant for an abnormal psychology class. This is one of the ways that graduate students put food on the table. I assumed this would mean making up and grading exams, and I was mortified when the professor casually mentioned that I would be giving several lectures to the class. This was a class of 400 students. I had taken a public speaking class in high school and I recalled being uncomfortable enough with ten people listening... I couldn't for the life of me imagine talking to 400 people.

The day of the first lecture approached, and I was about as anxious as I have ever been. I started to talk and I don't know that I made a great deal of sense, but to my surprise, no one jeered or fell asleep or left. I noticed that as the minutes went on, I became more and more comfortable... and after four or five lectures, I felt confident enough to tell some jokes and get people laughing and I even had a small sense of "working the crowd." I do a fair amount of speaking around the country now and generally really enjoy it... and I think this experience of pushing myself past what I thought I could comfortably do was the beginning for me.

The point of narratives like this is that doing what matters to us, even if it means being willing to experience something unpleasant or uncomfortable, puts us and our values in charge of our lives. In choosing to give the lectures, I was in charge of my life; anxiety was not in charge of my life.

The final practical element of a "willingness" approach to transcendence in spiritual care, as I think of it, is to suggest resources. In the reference section to this chapter, I have listed some ACT resources from New Harbinger for professionals and lay people. I don't get any commission for saying this, but I often suggest New Harbinger Publications (www.newharbinger.com) as a great resource for this particular subject and for other behavioral health issues. Based in Oakland, New Harbinger has been producing excellent behavioral health materials, much of it in hands-on, workbook formats, for over thirty years. The literacy level required of readers tends to be a little on the high side... perhaps "high school graduate" and above... but the material is empirically based and well written, and the prices are reasonable.

Mindfulness and Being Present

The third approach to transcendence in spiritual care conversations is mindfulness. Thanks largely to the pioneering efforts of Dr. Jon Kabat-Zinn to bring Eastern ideas about mindfulness to Western consciousness, this is a subject that is familiar to most of us who are clinicians in health and wellness care.

While the word "mindfulness" may signify particular meditative practices, mindfulness is foremost a way of relating to the world. Three elements of mindfulness are

- Paying attention, being aware
- In the present moment
- Without judgment, with acceptance

Paying attention and being aware are frequent themes in writing about spiritual life. Benedictine monk Brother David Steindl-Rast, for instance, speaks of being "awake" as a central feature of the spiritual life.[8] One can move through life asleep, distracted, preoccupied, or awake. To be awake means to deeply see and experience that which is there.

The ***present moment*** is important simply because it is all there is. The past may hold explanatory value in understanding how people arrived where they are. A consciousness about the future may, as we have discussed, provide direction and energy. But life is lived in present moments.

Non-judgment means accepting one's experience just as it is, without falling to the temptation of categorizing it as "good" or "bad." Many cultures have apocryphal tales similar to the story of the farmer who came upon an extraordinary gemstone in his field. Seeing his discovery, his neighbors unanimously congratulated him and said "that's wonderful." He replied, "Perhaps." Hearing the news, robbers broke into and ransacked his home, stealing the gemstone. His neighbors said, "That's terrible." He replied, "Perhaps." Drawing upon some savings, the farmer was able to restore and rebuild his home to be tidier and more comfortable than it had previously been. His neighbors said, "That's wonderful." He replied, "Perhaps." Seeing the improvement in the farmer's home, the local tax collector began demanding a larger tax payment. The farmer's neighbors said, "That's terrible." He replied, "Perhaps." His need for greater income to provide for the tax obligation led the farmer to experiment with a new crop, which he had not planted before and which turned out to yield a bountiful harvest. His neighbors said, "That's wonderful." The farmer replied, "Perhaps." And so forth.

Apart from the fact that the apocryphal farmer in such stories never seems like a particularly cheerful fellow who would be fun to have at your next office party, he does illustrate equanimity of spirit in just having his experiences be what they are, without judgment.

CLINICAL TIPS: Among the elements of mindfulness, I find that people particularly relate to the idea of the "present moment." Clinicians can develop this idea in two ways.

First, we may consider with patients the spiritual and emotional *costs* of living in the past or in the future.

- *Living in the past… focusing on the past… how does that work for you?*
- *As we have said, realistic future planning is fine, but when you dwell on what could happen in the future, as you are describing… what effect does that have on you?*
- *When you spend the time and spiritual energy you're describing to me on the past or the future, what does that keep you from doing?*
- *So… have there been times when you've missed out on something meaningful in life because you weren't really able to be "there" emotionally?*

The second way of developing the idea of the present moment is to consider with patients the *benefits* of being able to be present, here and now. Exploring with people when they have really felt "alive" or really "in tune with life" usually points to times when they have really been present to what was happening, here and now. Participating in the birth of a child. Being part of a team that pulls well together. Being caught up in the flow of discovering something new. Taking a new and milestone step in physical rehabilitation. Times like these of being really alive and engaged with life almost always relate to present moments.

A personal style of mine is that I also bring the idea of "present moment" into the conversations I have with patients.

With the two of us here, now, for instance, all we really have is the present moment. I have a history, like you do… growing up, what I've done for work, the kinds of relationships I've had with people. I have other things going on, other people I'm working with, other issues and decisions in the future for me… but any of those things that I focus on would take me away from really trying to understand you and listen to you and to be a part of your journey. So what I have to do… what I have to remind myself of… is to let go of all of that in order to really be here, now.

Clinicians may also suggest to patients that we can all exercise more control over present moments than we can over the unchangeable past or the uncertain future. I can't control what I did last Tuesday and I may or may not be able to control what will happen next Tuesday, but I can control whether or not I will be respectful or compassionate with you, now.

There are abundant resources for mindfulness. Jon Kabat-Zinn has published several books and ancillary products like CDs and collections of meditations. I often suggest the seminal book, *Wherever You Go, There You Are: Mindfulness Meditation in Everyday Life*,[9] originally published in the mid-nineties and available in subsequent editions. There are also thousands… millions, actually… of websites on the subject. For patients who are oriented to Internet learning, I usually suggest a Google search on "mindfulness Kabat-Zinn." This brings the search down to a more manageable 125,000, including a very good 75-minute YouTube video of Dr. Kabat-Zinn.

Non-attachment

A fourth approach to transcendence in spiritual care conversations is non-attachment. I include non-attachment on the list not because I have frequent conversations with people about it... I don't... but because it is an approach to transcendence and spiritual well-being that has ancient origins. Dating from the Sixth Century BCE, for instance, the Four Noble Truths of Buddhism hold that:

- Life entails suffering.
- Suffering is caused by attachment... our becoming emotionally and spiritually focused on craving what we want and don't want to happen.
- Suffering is overcome by foregoing attachment and cultivating a dispassionate approach to living in the present.
- The ongoing journey of spiritual self-improvement is charted by the Eightfold Path, of right intention, speech, action, livelihood and other expressions of ethical and personal development.

Suffering results from the attachment... modern sources often use the word, "craving..." to impermanent conditions such as wealth, prominence, power, and approval. Freedom from suffering comes from taking the non-attached and nonjudgmental perspective of the apocryphal farmer and putting energy and heart into developing present-moment compassion for others.

As I joked earlier, of course, the apocryphal farmer story is a pedagogical vehicle and is not meant to portray a real human response style. Non-attachment does not mean not caring, nor does it mean having no emotions. The woman I saw a couple of weeks ago whose daughter was killed in a motor vehicle accident was devastated, as I imagine any of us as parents would have been. The man I saw today whose beloved partner left to "find herself" was shocked and saddened. My wife and I were both teary this morning as we considered the stark decline of our ten-year-old golden retriever... legs collapsing, having great difficulty getting to his feet and walking... and what this might portend. These are not instances or pathological attachment; they are normal and honorable expressions of love.

CLINICAL TIPS: On some rare occasions, I have found the phrase, "non-attachment," popping up in conversations with patients, particularly those who bring some familiarity with Buddhism. More frequently, the *idea* of non-attachment... without necessarily using that language... comes up in conversations about the recurring theme of control. You can control the kind of person that you are going to be and how you live your life; you cannot control the results of your actions. Because you cannot control the results of your actions, you do well to be wary about being too attached to the results of your actions.

The man whose partner left may or may not at this point have much control about whether she will choose to return. He *can* choose to treat her with kindness, directness and respect. Much as he may wish his partner to return, he sets himself up for suffering if he becomes too preoccupied and attached to the outcome of her choosing to return. "Non-attachment," by contrast, means being able to be sad and wish that she would return, while investing his energy and heart into being the kind of person he wishes to be as he moves through this hard time.

Baseball addict that I am, I sometimes quote Red Sox designated hitter David Ortiz after he hit a game-winning home run against the Blue Jays in 2005:

Like I always say, you have to bring your "A" game... put a good swing on the ball and let things happen. If you go up there thinking about home runs, you're going to swing at all those pitches in the dirt.

This is good wisdom about non-attachment. The responsibility of the hitter is to "put a good swing on the ball" and then "let things happen." The hitter controls what he can control, and then takes a more dispassionate view of the outcome. Focusing on the outcome, moreover, makes the hitter more prone to swing at bad pitches and, paradoxically, makes the outcome less likely.

The clinical conversation, in other words, is to invite patients to exercise care in being too attached to outcomes that are beyond their control. Non-attachment as an approach to transcendence in spiritual care conversations, then, means to encourage patients to put energy and heart into being the kinds of people they wish to be, through the challenging circumstances that surround them.

Serenity

A fifth approach to transcendence in spiritual care conversations is serenity. The original use of the word "serene," in the early sixteenth century, pertained to calm and peaceful weather. More recently, the word has come to signify the same qualities of calmness and peacefulness in people, with the implication of having these qualities in the midst of the busyness and challenges of daily living.

Connors, Toscova and Tonigan provide an excellent conceptual review of serenity as applied to psychological and counseling settings.[10] Drawing on seminal earlier work by Roberts and Cunningham,[11] they summarize a number of key components of serenity, beginning with the abilities to find "detachment" and to cultivate an "inner haven" of peace and tranquility in the presence of external events and circumstances.

In the popular consciousness, serenity is very largely associated with the "Serenity Prayer." Drawing on 18th century roots, the Serenity Prayer was popularized in modern times by American Protestant theologian Reinhold Niebuhr and has been adopted widely in the 12-step movement.

Most frequently cited is the first stanza:

God grant me the serenity to accept things I cannot change,
The courage to change the things I can,
And the wisdom to know the difference.

The prayer continues:

Living one day at a time,
Enjoying one moment at a time,
Accepting hardship as a pathway to peace,
Taking this sinful world as it is,
Not as I would have it.

Trusting that you will make all things right
If I surrender to your will,
So that I may be reasonably happy in this life
And supremely happy with you forever in the next.

You will notice many of the themes that we have been considering:

- Letting go of circumstances beyond control
- Focusing attention and energy on aspects of life that are controllable
- Living in the present moment
- Being willing to experience the world as it is.

And the last stanza meshes with the 12-step emphasis of finding wisdom and being sustained in relationships with a Higher Power.

CLINICAL TIPS: My experience is that the idea of serenity comes up frequently with people who have been involved in Alcoholics Anonymous and other 12-step programs. I find that other people are also widely familiar with the Serenity Prayer, however, and that the distinction between what is and is not changeable is widely understood in that framework.

Clinically, the conversation often begins to explore what "serenity" means to patients and how they see it applying to their lives.

Clinician: *You mention "serenity..." what does that mean to you?*
Patient: *I was in AA years ago and we closed each meeting with the*

Serenity Prayer.

Clinician: *OK… and what does that mean to you now… what in the Serenity Prayer speaks to you?*

Patient: *Just the idea of accepting what you can't change and changing what you can.*

Clinician: *And how does that sort out for you… what you can't change and what you can change?*

Patient: *I'd love to work on bikes like I used to, but with my back I don't think I'm going to be able to.*

Clinician: *Motorcycles, right?*

Patient: *Yea… bikes, motorcycles*

Clinician: *Bikes… cool. So that's the part of serenity that you think you can't change?*

Patient: *Yea, I don't see that happening.*

Clinician: *OK, so say more about "serenity" around that… what does it mean to you to "accept" the fact that that isn't going to change?*

Patient: *Well, that's the hard part. It ain't easy, but somehow I know I've got to let go of a lot of stuff I used to do.*

Clinician: *Tell me about a time when you've been able to "accept" and "let go" a little bit… what is your sense about how you do that?*

The clinician goes on to pursue some of the questions and approaches from the conversational template we considered in the last chapter… clinician wisdom and patient wisdom about how to move toward "acceptance" and thinking collaboratively about possible next steps. The clinician also follows up on the second part of the Serenity Prayer… what it means to the patient to "change the things [he] can."

The conversation about the "changing what you can change" part of serenity can potentially touch on profoundly important spiritual issues. When former Superman actor Christopher Reeve was thrown from his horse in a riding accident in 1995, he suffered a spinal fracture that left him paralyzed from the shoulders down and needing ventilator assistance to breathe. As he realized the gravity of his condition, he wondered aloud if his family should just let him go, to which his wife responded, *"You're still you and I love you."[12]*

This quality of someone *being who they are* really touches on the core of the "changing what you can change" part of serenity, or perhaps more specifically the part of serenity having to do with acting with dignity on the choices that are available. Reeve didn't have a broad range of choices to make, but he did whatever he needed to do in order to express the essence of who he was as a person to his family. He expressed, we may assume, what was "vital and sacred" in terms of what it meant to him to love the people around him.

It always seems to me that it reflects wonderful spiritual design that the core choices that are left to us when much of the options of life are stripped away are also the choices that can touch on the qualities and values that we cherish most. Reeve didn't have much, but he could still choose to express love to his wife. Austrian psychiatrist Viktor Frankl didn't have much when he was in Theresienstadt concentration camp, but he could still encourage fellow prisoners. The patient from our practice who died of ALS a few weeks ago didn't have much, but he could still show glimpses of his trademark sense of humor. As House and Church point out,

> *The small truth is that you are sick today, or have PMS, or a cold, or feel feeble and weak. The Great Truth is that you are infinitely capable of doing good, thinking and saying kind words, and acting in loving and gentle ways.[13]* (p. 56)

Making choices that arise from cherished values makes for serenity. The clinical question is:

> *What is it that is most sacred and important to you in your life right now, given the choices that are available to you?*

We will explore clincial approaches to "valued directions" more thoroughly in the final part of this chapter.

Spiritual Surrender

Spiritual surrender, like non-attachment, is language that I almost never use in speaking with patients, but I include it in the list because it similarly is an approach to transcendence and spiritual well-being that has ancient origins. In their thorough and articulate recent review, Brenda Cole and Kenneth Pargament point out that surrender is described as a vital aspect of the spiritual life in writings as old as the Qur'an and the Bhagavad-Gita and as contemporary as the Course in Miracles.[14]

The modern scientific literature about spiritual surrender is largely associated with Pargament, who is professor of psychology at Bowling Green. Dr. Pargament has written extensively about religious coping, identifying and evaluating four predominant styles. In the *self-directing* approach, people pursue coping exclusively on their own initiative, having no reliance or involvement of God. In the *deferring* approach, people turn over challenging situations completely to God, exercising little or no personal responsibility on their own. In the *pleading* approach, people petition God to intervene on their behalf. Finally, in the *collaborative* approach, people pursue partnership relationships with God, turning to God for wisdom and sustaining, and also exercising their own initiative and creativity. It is perhaps not surprising that the collaborative approach is associated with better coping outcomes than the others.

Spiritual surrender is a collaborative approach. Spiritual surrender items on Pargament's religious coping scales, as examples, are:

- Did my best and then turned the situation over to God
- Did what I could and then put the rest in God's hands
- Took control over what I could and gave the rest up to God[15]

In locating spiritual surrender within the rubric of religious coping, however, Cole and Pargament emphasize that spiritual surrender is more than just a coping approach. Spiritual surrender is not a tool by which to engineer good outcomes, even though it may indeed be associated with better coping outcomes. Rather, they argue, spiritual surrender is fundamentally an expression of spiritual life and commitment:

> *Through spiritual surrender, control is abandoned for the sake of the sacred, be it transcendent purpose, ideal, relationship, or commitment.*

CLINICAL TIPS: This is another approach to transcendence in spiritual care conversations that I will pursue if patients mention it first. If the language and framework of "spiritual surrender" is part of the experience of the patient, then I will pursue this with the same kind of exploratory conversation we have considered before:

- *What does "spiritual surrender" mean to you?*
- *When has this been helpful or significant in your life?*
- *What would "spiritual surrender" mean in terms of where you go from here?*

Introducing the idea of surrender in conversations seems to me to be more in the province of spiritual care specialists.

Gratitude and gratefulness

The seventh approach to transcendence in spiritual care conversations is gratitude. A middle aged man with end-stage colon cancer reflects,

> *This may sound strange, but I have come to believe that cancer has been the worst thing that ever happened in my life and also the best thing that ever happened in my life. Before my illness, I was going along, doing what I do, but with my cancer, I've really felt much more of a sense of delight in life than I ever had before. I think I used to emotionally look forward to things in the future that I thought would make me happy, but I realize now that the real delight is just in opening my heart to what is unfolding in my life right now... being able to be*

grateful for the moments of my life as I experience them, one by one.

For this man, the ability to experience "delight" and "grate-fulness" was a vital source of aliveness and transcendence in the midst of an illness from which he was to die in three or four months.

The practice of gratitude or gratefulness reflects ancient spiritual wisdom. In the Judaic tradition, the sacred texts… Psalms being a rich example… are replete with expressions of thanksgiving to God. In the Islamic tradition, the daily practice of *Salat,* or prayer, focuses the worshipper in a relationship of adoration and gratitude to God. In the Christian tradition, Paul of Tarsus instructs the church in Thessalonica to be "thankful in all circumstances, for this is God's will for you."

In all of these traditions, gratitude is not a situation-specific thankfulness… as you would say "thanks" when someone hands you a cup of coffee… it is a spiritual practice and an attitude toward daily living. Paul instructs followers not just to be thankful in circumstances that they would consider "good," but in *all* cir-cumstances. The spiritual underpinning of this practice is that an attitude of gratefulness helps people to be open to the creative and healing movement of God even in challenging circumstances. For the man with colon cancer, the practice of delight and grate-fulness… amid the ravages of his illness… allowed him to expe-rience joy in the moments of his daily living that he had not expe-rienced before.

The practice of gratitude or gratefulness also is a subject of current empirical inquiry. Much of this work has been led by Dr. Robert Emmons, who is a professor of psychology at the Uni-versity of California, Davis. With several colleagues, Emmons has instructed research subjects in educational and clinical settings to keep weekly and daily journals of gratitude.[16] Compared with subjects who monitored daily hassles or neutral events, the people in these studies who kept gratitude journals experienced a variety of beneficial outcomes, including enhanced mood, fewer physical symptoms, greater self-care and goal attainment, greater sense of connectedness to others, and higher optimism. If you are interested in pursuing the empirical literature in greater detail, you can go to Google, type in "Emmons gratitude" and enjoy perusing the 66,000 hits. His body of work, by the way, includes approaches to the measurement of gratefulness and studies of gratefulness as a disposition, as well as intervention studies about gratitude practices.

My own perspective is that gratitude begins with wonder. Being grateful starts with being awake to the little and big things in life that are wonderful, amazing, surprising, and often somewhat mysterious. The way your body knows how to deal with a laceration so that a week or two later, there is no trace of it ever having been there. The way your one year old daughter stumbles and crawls one day and walks the next. The way you can pay the postal service 42 cents to deliver a letter to Uncle Dean in Colby, Kansas, and you can bet the farm that it will get there. The way the same pair of mallards (so I assume, anyway) make their way to my vernal pond when they migrate back to Maine in the spring. The way your post-stroke patient manages to live life with dignity and grace in spite of apraxia of speech.

A discipline or practice of gratitude, moreover… in keeping with the spiritual traditions we have touched upon… extends not only to smelling the proverbial flowers along the path, but also to the circumstances that we typically define as more challenging. A colleague recently commented that URI symptoms like coughing, runny nose, and fever… which we typically think of as signs of ill-health… are really better understood as positive signs of good health. Reacting to an incursion of viral critters with the processes of a respiratory tract infection is just the way that healthy, well-functioning bodies are supposed to react.

Similarly, it seems to me increasingly that some of the emotional experiences that we address as clinicians really can be understood as wonderful expressions of the ways that human spirits are supposed to work. We typically think of "anxiety" and "depression" as "symptoms" that need to be cured, but there is a sense in which they can also be understood as wonderful (albeit uncomfortable) signals that something in life needs to change. I believe more and more, for instance, that anxiety is a signal that is hard wired (evolutionarily or by design) to point the way toward growth. If we are anxious about driving, leaving the house, expressing anger, or telling someone we love them, anxiety points the way to experiences that can help to expand the scope of our lives. I frequently suggest to patients, therefore, to *do what makes you anxious; don't do what makes you depressed."* There are limits, of course; anxiety about bungee-jumping off of Royal Gorge is a healthy signal of another sort; it is octagonal and red.

Jeanne House and Dawson Church have written an excellent recent chapter that develops further the idea of "symptoms as signals" in the context of spirituality and health.[13]

A particularly remarkable body of work about gratefulness and wonder comes from Brother David Steindl-Rast. Brother David is an Austrian-born American Benedictine monk who has been engaged in inter-religious dialogue, spiritual renewal, and peace initiatives for many years. He is the author of several books about gratefulness,[8] silence, and shared spiritual experience. He is also the initiator of an extraordinary website about gratefulness, appropriately named www.gratefulness.org. The website has stories, resources, e-cards, a virtual labyrinth and a virtual candle-lighting exercise. Very nice.

CLINICAL TIPS: Two simple but powerful exercise from the positive psychology movement are "three good things" and the "gratitude visit."[17] The former invites people to write three things that went well and their causes each day for a week. The purpose is both to encourage people to track positive events, for which they may be grateful, and to encourage them to consider ways that they may have been responsible for these events.

The gratitude visit is particularly intriguing. This exercise invites people to write a letter to someone who has been meaningful in their life but whom they have not properly thanked, then to deliver it in person. As you may envision, Seligman and colleagues report profoundly touching stories of people's experiences with this exercise.

I find that patients frequently raise the issue of gratitude, or at least or putting their situations in perspective by thanking their lucky stars that they're not worse. Part of the clinical approach to gratefulness is to take what patients say and invite them to consider gratefulness in a broader way.

Clinician: *So you were on the mental health inpatient unit for three or four days last week... how was that for you?*
Patient: *Pretty good.*
Clinician: *What was it in particular that was helpful for you?*
Patient: *I think just seeing some of the other people there... I'm thankful that I'm not that bad off. Some people who just stared into space and one guy who was just chanting and jabbering all day long.*
Clinician: *Wow. When you use the word "thankful," tell me more about thankfulness and how thankfulness fits into your life...*

If people are interested in pursuing a practice of gratitude, I most often suggest one or two among three approaches. First, I invite people to keep a daily gratitude journal in whatever way feels comfortable for them. I emphasize that the daily practice is important and that gratitude for "small" experiences like the car starting is just as important as gratitude for "larger" experiences like getting a promotion at work. Second, I refer patients who are Internet-connected to gratefulness.org. Third, I point out that there are a large number of popular press books about the practice of gratitude, and I invite patients who are so inclined to spend a little time in their local bookseller seeing what may inspire them.

Forgiveness

The final approach to transcendence in spiritual care conversations that I will mention is forgiveness.

One of the most striking images I have ever seen is the photograph of Pope John Paul II meeting with his would-be assassin, Turkish terrorist Mehmet Ali Agca, in Agca's prison cell in Rome. The two of them sit facing each other in the far corner of a bare room, the Pope speaking and Agca listening intently. A Turkish terrorist who believed that the Pope incarnated the evils of the capitalist world, Acga had shot and wounded him two years earlier. Now John Paul was coming to Acga "as a brother whom I have pardoned." The prison visit and John Paul's subsequent meetings with Acga's family apparently moved his assailant deeply; Acga wrote the Pope wishing him well during his final illness and grieved for his loss when he died in 2005.

More than the fact that the Pope's visit had a transforming effect on his assailant, I think I am touched by John Paul's courage and spiritual integrity in coming to Acga as he did... "as a brother," bearing a message of forgiveness. The Pope presumably had no guarantee of what Acga's reaction might be, but he apparently chose the path of forgiveness because it was important to him, regardless of the outcome.

So it is with forgiveness; it is a commitment and path that is followed by wounded people for their own reasons, and which may or may not result in apology or reconciliation with offenders. Forgiveness is a form of transcendence because it frees people from the potential bitterness, hatred, and immobilization of having been wounded.

Forgiveness is another ancient practice with a burgeoning modern empirical literature. In the United States, there have been three particularly active centers of research and initiatives in forgiveness, in Wisconsin, Virginia, and California.

Robert Enright, PhD at the University of Wisconsin-Madison is the founder of the International Forgiveness Institute, a center for research, education, and community since the mid-nineties.[18] With his wife, he has also developed a forgiveness curriculum for young children which has been integrated with promising results in school systems in Belfast, Northern Ireland and in inner-city Milwaukee.[19]

Enright's "process model" of forgiveness involves 20 steps that cluster into four phases:[20]

- An *uncovering* phase involves recognizing and confronting anger and other negative emotions associated with mistreatment from another person.
- A *decision* phase involves a choice by the injured individual… often arising out of the recognition that change needs to happen in order to bring about healing… to take preliminary steps in the direction of forgiveness, such as forgoing thoughts and intentions of revenge.
- A *work* phase involves exploring new ways to think about the injurer and understanding the forces that influenced him or her. The work of this understanding often results in some sense of compassion or empathy toward the injurer; it may or may not result in reconciliation. The work phase also involves acceptance of the pain of the injury and choosing not to pass it on to others.
- An *outcome and deepening* phase involves greater emotional healing and often a discovery or creation of meaning and purpose from the injury and the healing process.

Based at Virginia Commonwealth University, Everett L. Worthington, Jr., PhD is the Executive Director of A Campaign for Forgiveness Research. A prolific researcher and researcher, Worthington knows whereof he speaks; his mother was brutally murdered by an intruder and he has drawn upon his professional work in forgiveness in his own life.

Worthington proposes a five-step "pyramid model" of forgiveness with the acronym REACH:[21, 22]

- **R**ecall the hurt
- **E**mpathize with the injurer
- **E**xtend an **A**ltruistic gesture or gift of forgiveness

- Acknowledge forgiving intention: make a public **Com**mitment to forgive
- **H**old on to forgiveness as it is challenged by reminders of the injury

The process of forgiveness, for Worthington, is aimed at personal peace and wholeness, with substantial attention to the possibility of restored relationships. A great deal of resource material is available at his VCU website, http://www.people.vcu.edu/~eworth/. This includes participant and leader manuals for forgiveness groups (for both secular groups and groups tailored toward Christian faith) and participant and leader manuals for groups of couples, emphasizing forgiveness and reconciliation.

Frederic Luskin, PhD (may I point out that he spells "Frederic" the correct way) is the director of the Stanford Forgiveness Projects, another nationally prominent center for research, education and community initiatives. The work that Luskin and colleagues have done applying forgiveness principles with traumatized populations in Northern Ireland, Sierra Leone, and from the 9/11 attacks is particularly compelling. The Northern Ireland projects, for instance, have involved bringing together Catholic and Protestant people who have had loved ones murdered in the sectarian violence and inviting them to explore specific approaches to forgiving the people who had perpetrated the murders.

Luskin's paradigm for forgiveness includes nine steps.[23] It suggests that the ongoing distress from undeserved injuries is associated more with *painful thoughts and emotions about those injuries* than it is with the injuries themselves. It proposes that people let go of "unenforceable rules" about how other people should behave and to recognize that happiness and well-being come from putting energy in positive directions toward meaningful life goals. Moving through these steps toward forgiveness, Luskin says, is a "heroic choice" that helps people to restore "personal power" on behalf of life lived well.[24]

With some differences in specifics, these three approaches share some common features. They all emphasize:

- Forgiveness is *unilateral*... having to do with letting go of emotions and distress from mistreatment, and choosing to invest energy in meaningful living. *Reconciliation* is bilateral... when injurers choose to join in the process of acknowledging the reality of the injury and pursuing a restoration of relationship.
- Forgiveness must be grounded in *acknowledgment of feelings* associated with mistreatment and injuries.
- Forgiveness is a *process* of working through mistreatment; it is not a snap or shallow decision.
- Forgiveness typically involves *coming to see injurers in a new light,* with intellectual understanding and often with empathy.
- Forgiveness is *paradoxical;* by extending forgiveness to other people, we promote our own healing.

I should point out, by the way, that Americans certainly don't have a corner on the market with forgiveness. There have been some extraordinary international initiatives. More than a dozen countries, for instance, have established truth and reconciliation commissions for the purposes of establishing the facts about periods of national strife and destruction, and offering degrees of amnesty and reconciliation for people who come forward as victims or as abusers. The prototypical example of a "TRC" is in South Africa, where the truth and reconciliation process is generally credited with having helped substantially to restore individual dignity and social order in the wake of decades of oppression and violence.[25]

Another extraordinary initiative is based at Coventry in the United Kingdom. An industrial city that was key to Britain's military efforts in World War II, Coventry was fire-bombed in 1940, with the loss of 60,000 buildings and several hundred lives. Beholding the destruction of the irreplaceable 12th century cathedral, the cathedral Provost immediately urged his community to banish thoughts of revenge and set in motion a process of forgiveness, reconciliation, and partnership with other international cities (including Dresden, in Germany) that had suffered the same fate. Today, Coventry University hosts a Centre for Peace and Reconciliation Studies that builds on the mission of forgiveness that began over half a century ago.[26]

CLINICAL TIPS: As much as any of these approaches to transcendence, thorough explorations of forgiveness will frequently fall in the domain of spiritual care professionals. Having said that, I think there are a number of approaches and principles for providers of health and wellness care that can begin to point toward and draw upon the healing power of forgiveness.

Count the cost. Clinicians can help to establish with patients whether there is a significant cost associated with holding on to bitterness and resent.

Clinician: *So you're saying that your son has taken advantage of you with not repaying the two loans and then with the real estate transaction?*
Patient: *That and a lifetime of lying.*
Clinician: *Wow, I can imagine... and how is that for you?*
Patient: *It stinks... I haven't been perfect, but I've tried to be a good dad and this is what I've always gotten.*
Clinician: *When you say, "It stinks," say more about how this affects you...*
Patient: *I just get really angry... bitter...*
Clinician: *And when you say, "bitter," how does that affect you?*
Patient: *That's probably why I'm here... high blood pressure, can't sleep...*
Clinician: *So if you stay bitter, it sounds like things won't be going in a good direction for you.*
Patient: *That's for sure.*

Clinician: *So… what's your sense about what the alternative is to staying bitter?*
Patient: *My wife says I need to forgive him and move on.*
Clinician: *And what are your thoughts about that?*

Allow patients to make the choices they need to make. I would not presume that forgiveness is the right approach for anybody. I happen to think that it is a pretty good approach to transcendence, and there are solid data from Enright, Worthington, Luskin and others, but the choice whether to forgive rests with patients and not with me. I believe that an approach of honoring people thinking through the choices that are best for them is preferable to trying to sell someone on forgiveness. This is analogous to the motivational interviewing literature, which suggests that patients are often better served by clinicians earnestly pursuing with them the advantages and disadvantages of smoking, rather than just telling them that they should stop.

Work with stages of change. Another helpful approach from the motivational interviewing literature is the stages of change framework. Developed by psychologist James Prochaska, the framework posits that people fall on a continuum in terms of their readiness to make changes, from "precontemplation" to "action," with intermediate steps along the way.[27, 28] The clinical significance is that clinicians devote more energy on the issue of "why change" with patients who are earlier in the stages of change process, and devote more energy to the issue of "how change" as people move closer to action.

With the patient who is bitter about his son, relatively early in stages of change:

Patient: *My wife says I need to forgive him and move on.*
Clinician: *And what are your thoughts about that?*
Patient: *I think she's nuts… I'm no way going to forgive him and let him get away with all he's done.*

Clinician: *Are "letting him get away with it" and "forgiveness" the same?*

Patient: *Aren't they?*

Clinician: *I guess it depends on what "forgiveness" means... how would you put into words what that means to you?*

Patient: *Let them go ahead and do whatever they want.*

Clinician: *OK... I can see that wouldn't make forgiveness very appealing when your wife mentions that to you. Since you raised the topic of forgiveness, can I toss out a couple of ideas?*

Patient: *OK*

Clinician: *When most people write about forgiveness, they pretty much say that the people who mistreat you still have consequences for what they do, even if you forgive them... the Pope forgave that guy who shot him, for instance, but the guy is still in jail for life. The other thing is that we hear from people who write about forgiveness is that forgiveness is fundamentally about letting go of bitterness and resent and being able to get on with life... whether or not the people who cause injury ever change... which might be relevant for you, since you're telling me how much bitterness affects you.*

Patient: *How can you let go of being bitter if people who hurt you are still out there pulling the same stunts they've always done?*

Clinician: *That's right... that's the idea... letting it go even if people don't change. Your question is great... how do you do that? Is that something you'd be interested in looking into some more? I could give you some reading, or we could talk more, or I could suggest a chaplain who works with us who is very helpful with people around these issues.*

Patient: *Let me think about it.*

With the patient who is bitter about his son, relatively farther along in stages of change:

Patient: *My wife says I need to forgive him and move on.*

Clinician: *And what are your thoughts about that?*

Patient: *I think she's right.*

Clinician: *Say more…*

Patient: *Somehow I do need to get over this… it's eating me up. Susan says she forgives our son and I probably need to be working on that, too.*

Clinician: *How do you do that?*

Patient: *I need to figure that out… it's easy for Susan.*

Clinician: *Is that something you'd be interested in looking into some more? I could give you some reading, or we could talk more, or I could suggest a chaplain who works with us who is very helpful with people around these issues.*

Patient: *I know someone who met with the chaplain and said that was real helpful… so that would be available for me?*

Tell stories. Stories, in general, are powerful ways of communicating ideas to patients. With forgiveness, in particular, the feeling of the concepts and theories often pales in comparison with real stories of human experience.

Driving home late one night, a young man was killed in an automobile crash with a drunk driver. The blood alcohol level of the drunk driver… a young man about the same age… was twice the legal limit. The driver had just left a bar and was driving on the wrong side of the road with headlights off.

The young man who died was a real all-star… president of his high school student body, captain of the football team… destined for great things. The driver had had several previous brushes with the law and was driving with a suspended license.

The death was devastating for the parents. They lay awake nights for weeks after the accident, nursing feelings of loss and fury and revenge. Then one night, the mother was struggling to go back to sleep when she heard a voice saying, "I don't want you to be like this." She took this seriously and came to believe that this was a serious invitation for her to change direction in how she had been reacting to her son's tragic death.

The first step in her change of direction was to wonder what life experiences had brought the young driver to the point where he had had the legal and substance abuse problems she knew about. She thought... correctly as it turned out... that he must have had a sad or abusive time growing up. She reflected later that this exercise didn't make her want to excuse the driver, but helped her to see him as a little bit more human... and as she did that, she noticed her own feelings of fury and revenge starting to calm.

She attended the court hearings and trial of the young driver, who for the most part sat in an impassive way. She resisted the idea of speaking with him, but she did draft a letter telling about her son and describing some of her own struggles with his death. She concluded the letter by saying that she didn't know what the young driver's life had been like, but she saw that he was being profoundly hurt by the accident and its aftermath, as well... and she hoped that he might somehow find some good coming to his life out of everything that was happening. She debated for a couple of weeks whether she should send the letter, and eventually did.

Some time later, the mother received back a response from the young driver's mother. It said that her son had always been troubled and didn't have any interest in corresponding, but that she herself so much appreciated the letter that her son had shown her and wondered if the mother of the boy who died would be so kind as to get together at some point.

The two mothers did indeed meet and struck up a friendship that led to their developing a program together in which they speak in high schools about loss and forgiveness.

The father of the young man who died was not so fortunate. He was never able to let go of his bitterness and vengeful feelings, descending himself into alcohol abuse and dying of a massive heart attack at age 54.

Suggest resources. For people who are interested in exploring the possibilities of forgiveness further, I have a collection of resources that I recommend. Enright, Worthington, and Luskin all have popular-press, readily-accessible books about their work and perspectives. I also suggest an excellent book that dates from the very early years of the modern renewal of interest in forgiveness, but remains current and is now available in an updated version, *Forgive and Forget: Healing the Hurts We Don't Deserve*, by Fuller Theological Seminary emeritus professor Lewis B. Smedes.[29]

Collaborate with spiritual care professionals. Finally, I can underscore the substantial role that our spiritual care colleagues play in a detailed exploration of forgiveness and some of the other approaches to transcendence that we have considered. It pays to get to know the chaplains, spiritual directors, and clergy in your community… or at least a manageable subset of them… for purposes of drawing upon the expertise and time that they can offer.

STRATEGY 17
Experiment with one or
two approaches to transcendence

You have read (or perused) a lot of material about eight approaches to transcendence. Pick out one or two that particularly resonate with you and experiment with how you can bring them into conversations where patients need to transcend life experiences that are holding them back.

ENCOURAGING PATIENTS
IN VALUED DIRECTIONS

You will recall Joanne, the nursing student at the beginning of this chapter, saying that "I couldn't bring my friend back or change any of what's happened or make my lupus go away, but I could make my life count from here on." Her eloquent comment touches on both of the focal points of this chapter, transcendence and valued directions.

As I suggested earlier, transcendence and the pursuit of valued directions go together. They are complementary. They need each other. Meaningful living needs transcendence; Joanne can't really commit her heart and energy to moving in valued directions without making peace with her losses and her illness. Just as much, transcendence needs the pursuit of valued directions; Joanne's making peace with the unchangeable elements of her life would be a hollow exercise unless she uses the freedom that transcendence provides to "make my life count from here on."

To this point in the chapter, we have considered a variety of approaches to transcendence. Now we look at the matching piece, encouraging patients in valued directions.

I should point out that we have already considered this subject in some detail. In Chapter Six, we reviewed literature and approaches to cultivating personal strengths and positive qualities of character. I suggested a number of conversational approaches to exploring personal values, which are equally applicable to patients as they are to caregivers:

- *What do you particularly take pride in with regard to how you try to live your life day to day? What kind of person do you try to be?*
- *When have there been times when you have really felt positive about what you were doing? What memorable events do you recall that felt good emotionally and spiritually? What qualities of character are visible in these events?*
- *How do you want to be living and handling the challenging situations that come your way?*
- *When are the times when you feel like you are really connecting with a patient, friend, or family member?*
- *When are the times when your energy or spirit brings a little light or goodness into the world?*
- *When are the times when you are really giving life to your calling or vocation?*
- *Recalling Howard Thurman's comment, what does it mean to you to "come alive" and when/how does this happen?*

- *If you were planning to move to Millinocket, Maine and had a going-away gathering of your friends and associates, what would you hope and expect they would say about you?* (In Chapter Six, I said "Bozeman, Montana", but I want to be fair and acknowledge that to a lot of readers, *my* neighborhood it at the end of the earth.)

Related to the Bozeman/Millinocket question, by the way, is the "deathbed" question from the Positive Psychology literature.[30] The deathbed question simply involves picturing that final stage of life and to envision, looking back over the years, what you would want to have spent more time doing.

Such questions can be helpful conversation starters… or helpful questions to move conversations along… in inviting patients to think about what makes life meaningful for them.

In Chapter Six, we also considered some structured approaches to defining personal values and qualities of character. These approaches included the "VIA Signature Strengths Questionnaire" (available at www.authentichappiness.org) and the great "sortable" list of personal values from Dr. William Miller at the University of New Mexico (http://motivationalinterview.org/library/values-cardsort.pdf).

In Chapter Nine, we explored a number of approaches to helping patients define and pursue meaningful goals in the framework of the template for spiritual care conversations. In considering the "What matters to you and where do you want to go?" part of the template, we looked at ways of helping patients to identify values that arise out of what is "vital and sacred" for them. You may wish to refer back to these sections.

At this point, I want to suggest an additional perspective on developing and pursuing values; a coherent exploration of values as they relate to personal roles. My thinking about this began in 1982 with the publication of the journal article that I suspect I have recommended more than any other single article over the years, Eric

Cassell's commentary in the New England Journal of Medicine on "The Nature of Suffering and the Goals of Medicine."[31]

Dr. Cassell argues that suffering is different from physical distress. Physical distress arises from somatic experiences, while suffering arises out of the personal meaning and significance of those experiences. You and I could perhaps find ourselves with the physical distress and mobility limitations of a severe ankle sprain. For you, the suffering might be modest or negligible… if, for instance, having an ankle sprain gives you the opportunity to slow down, drink tea and read books more than you are typically able to do. For me, the suffering is substantial, because I know from unfortunate past episodes that I am beginning a sentence of six weeks of not being able to play basketball.

Cassell says that suffering is experienced when the intactness of persons is compromised. A useful way of thinking about our intactness or integrity as persons, moreover, is to look at our role relationships. I am a psychologist. I am a medical educator. I am a colleague. I am a husband, father, and father-in-law. I am a neighbor and an advocate for some causes in my community. I am a friend. I am a basketball player and a member of a community of men who have played together for a long time. I am a fiddler and a member of a community of musicians who come together regularly for the joy of making music and occasionally, to perform. And more.

For each of these role relationships, suffering may be experienced in particular ways arising out of physical distress. A back injury may affect one's role as a backhoe operator, but not much affect one's role as a caring sibling.

Roles link uniquely to suffering, and roles also link uniquely to values. In the same way that our suffering is marked by the disruption of meaningful roles, our emotional and spiritual wellness is marked by the engagement in meaningful roles.

A coherent way to encourage patients in pursuing valued directions, therefore, is to invite them to define and focus on values in the key roles of their lives.

STRATEGY 18

Invite patients to define key role values

Ask patients to list some key roles in their lives… family roles, work roles, community roles, recreational roles, and so forth. My experience is that we explain the concept, give patients a few examples (as I have done a few paragraphs ago) and have them take it away.

Having listed key roles, patients then are asked to put into words their values about each of those roles, considering questions such as:

- *What is most important to you about this role?*
- *How do you want to be approaching this role?*
- *What would tell you that you are pursuing this role well?*

Then, as patients define values for their key roles, the next questions are where they see themselves with these values now, and what they might do to move closer to the ways they wish to be.

I get interesting responses from this exercise. Some are elegant in simplicity, such as the woman whose statement of values about her role as a parent was to "love my children and be honest with them."

Some responses are more elaborate and can be charming in different ways. A middle aged man defined his recreational roles and life largely in terms of playing softball. Listing values for this particular role in his life, he wrote a note saying:

You always run the ball out. You always hustle. You take pride in your work. You never show up your opponents if you happen to find yourself coming out ahead. You stay cool and keep your dignity when you fail. You respect and encourage your teammates. You respect and encourage your opponents. You play your game, not somebody else's.

My presumption is that his faithfully following these values will enhance the quality and richness of that corner of his life.

SUMMARY

- Transcendence and the pursuit of valued directions are recurrent themes in spiritual care.
- Transcendence does not mean avoidance or distraction from pain: rather, it has to do with the journey of letting go or making peace with the unchangeable elements of life.
- We reviewed eight frameworks, with clinical tips, for supporting people with transcendence:
  - Letting go
  - Willingness/acceptance
  - Mindfulness and being present
  - Non-attachment
  - Serenity
  - Spiritual surrender
  - Gratitude and gratefulness
  - Forgiveness
- The pursuit of valued directions... making meaningful life choices and finding meaningful life paths... arises out of transcendence and gives meaning to transcendence. Spiritual care encourages patients in the interwoven process of letting go and moving forward.
- We have explored a number of approaches to identifying and pursuing valued directions, including
  - Conversational and structured approaches to cultivating personal strengths and positive qualities of character (Chapter 6)
  - Defining and pursuing meaningful goals in the framework of the template for spiritual care conversations (Chapter 9)
  - Inviting patients to define values associated with the key roles of their lives.

Joanne the nursing student, by the way, was last seen working at a county hospital and volunteering at a free clinic in a large city... and saying that she had never been happier. Letting go and making her life count, indeed.

REFERENCES

1. Hamilton K, Murphy J. *The H.O.P.E. Story*. South Paris, ME: HOPE Healing Publications; 2007.

2. Hamilton K. *SoulCircling: The Journey to the Who*. South Paris, ME: HOPE Healing Publications; 2002.

3. Hayes S, Strosahl K, Wilson K. *Acceptance and Commitment Therapy: An Experiential Approach to Behavior Change*. New York: Guilford; 2003.

4. Hayes S, Smith S. *Get Out of Your Mind and Into Your Life*. Oakland, CA: New Harbinger; 2005.

5. Eifert G, Forsyth J, Hayes S. *Acceptance & Commitment Therapy for Anxiety Disorders: A Practitioner's Treatment Guide to Using Mindfulness, Acceptance, and Values-Based Behavior Change Strategies*. Oakland, CA: New Harbinger; 2005.

6. Lejeune C. *The Worry Trap: How to Free Yourself from Worry & Anxiety using Acceptance and Commitment Therapy*. Oakland, CA: New Harbinger; 2007.

7. Dahl J, Wilson K, Luciano C, Hayes S. *Acceptance and Commitment Therapy for Chronic Pain*. Reno, NV: Context; 2005.

8. Steindl-Rast D. *Gratefulness, The Heart of Prayer: An Approach to Life in Fullness*. Mahwah, NJ: Paulist Press; 1984.

9. Kabat-Zinn J. *Wherever You Go, There You Are: Mindfulness Meditation in Everyday Life*. New York: Hyperion; 2005.

10. Connors G, Toscova R, Tonigan J. Serenity. In: Miller W, ed. *Integrating Spirituality into Treatment: Resources for Practitioners*. Washington, DC: American Psychological Association; 1999.

11. Roberts K, Cunningham G. Serenity: Concept analysis and measurement. *Educ Gerontology*. 1990;16:577-589.

12. Younis S. Biography. Available at: http://www.chrisreevehomepage.com/biography.html.

13. House J, Church D. Signals of the soul. In: Church D, ed. *Healing the Heart of the World*. Santa Rosa, CA: Elite; 2005.

14. Cole B, Pargament K. Spiritual surrender: A paradoxical path to control. In: Miller W, ed. *Integrating Spirituality into Treatment: Resources for Practitioners*. Washington, DC: American Psychological Association; 1999.

15. Pargament K, Koenig H, Perez L. The many methods of religious coping: development and initial validation of the RCOPE. *J Clin Psychol.* 2000;56(4):519-543.

16. Emmons R, McCullough M. Counting blessings versus burdens: Experimental studies of gratitude and subjective well-being in daily life. *J Pers Soc Psych.* 2003;84:377-389.

17. Seligman M, Steen T, Park N, Peterson C. Positive psychology progress: Empirical validation of interventions. *Am Psychol.* 2005;60(5):410-421.

18. Enright R. *Forgiveness Is a Choice: A Step-By-Step Process for Resolving Anger and Restoring Hope.* Washington, DC: American Psychological Association; 2001.

19. Hill K. Robert Enright: Planting seeds of forgiveness in Belfast and Milwaukee. Available at: http://www.wisconsinidea.wisc.edu/profiles/Enright/.

20. Enright R, Reed G. Process Model. Available at: http://www.forgiveness-institute.org/html/process_model.htm. Accessed 2009.

21. Worthington E. *Five Steps to Forgiveness: The Art and Science of Forgiving: Bridges to Wholeness and Hope*: Crown; 2001.

22. Worthington E. *Forgiving and Reconciling: Bridges to Wholeness and Hope.* Downers Grove, IL: InterVarsity Press; 2003.

23. Luskin F. *Forgive for Good; A Proven Prescription for Health and Happiness.* New York: HarperCollins; 2003.

24. Luskin F. Nine steps to forgiveness. Available at: http://www.learningtoforgive.com/steps.htm. Accessed 2009.

25. Mokushane T. Truth and Reconciliation Commission Website. Available at: http://www.doj.gov.za/trc/, 2009.

26. Rigby R. Centre for Peace and Reconciliation Studies. Available at: http://www.coventry.ac.uk/researchnet/peacestudies/a/865, 2009.

27. Prochaska J, DiClemente C, Norcross J. In search of how people change. *Am Psychol.* 1992;47:1102-1104.

28. Zimmerman G, Olsen C, Bosworth M. A 'Stages of Change' Approach to Helping Patients Change Behavior. *Am Fam Phys.* 2000;61(5):1409-1416.

29. Smedes L. *Forgive and Forget: Healing the Hurts We Don't Deserve.* New York: HarperOne; 2007.

30. Peterson C, Seligman M. *Character Strengths and Virtues.* Oxford/New York: Oxford/APA; 2004.

31. Cassell E. The nature of suffering and the goals of medicine. *NEJM*. 1982;306(11):639-645.

ORGANIZATIONAL: CONNECTING WITH THE SHARED ENERGY OF PEOPLE WORKING TOGETHER

In the last six chapters, we have explored the *personal* arena of spiritual care… the importance of cultivating our own centeredness, intention and presence… and the *clinical* arena of spiritual care… helping patients to identify and give expression to the things that are "vital and sacred" in their lives.

In the final section of spiritual care approaches, we turn our attention to the *organizational* arena. As I have suggested earlier, organizations have souls. The phenomenon of "soul," in the context of organizational life, goes a variety of names; "spirit," "atmosphere," "culture," "tone," "environment," and so forth. Some organizations have it; some do not, and the difference is usually palpable.

There is, as I have also described, some substantial literature about organizational soul (by its various names) in health care. In Chapter 4, we reviewed data from cross-sectional studies of organizational culture, intervention research and transformational narratives, and studies of exemplary practices that attest to the fact that organizational soul matters. Health care organizations that cultivate soul… a shared sense of mission, respect, and empowerment of employees, a spirit of community and caring among workers… do better than organizations that do not with respect to employee retention and satisfaction, patient satisfaction, performance improvement and process measures, and health care outcomes. Organizational soul, in other words, is not a soft and superfluous nicety; it is central to doing what we do.

Exploration and writing about organizational culture and soul in the business sector, in fact, goes back for decades. Dating from the 1990s, there have been a flurry of business books, representing some substantial management research, exploring qualities of "soul" and even "spirituality" in the workplace.[1-8] Being a practical guy, I am not so much interested in writing a review of this literature as I am considering with you the question of how the soul of organizations may be nurtured as part of the overall process of spiritual care.

The next three chapters, then, will look at some specific approaches to developing and nurturing organizational mission and values (Chapter 11), cultivating a spirit of community (Chapter 12), and fostering empowering health care leadership (Chapter 13).

## Chapter Eleven

Honor Organizational Mission and Values

There is no power for change greater than a community discovering what it cares about.[9]

Margaret Wheatley

A Tale of Two Cities:

Our hospital did well, at least in terms of patient care and what it felt like to be working there, when it was locally owned. Two or three years ago, it was bought out by a national for-profit corporation and it totally changed. They brought in a new CEO, a business-type, who is really just concerned about the bottom line and has an unbearable top-down management style. She introduced herself to us by making the hospital more "efficient" by firing half a dozen senior long-term employees who had really been the heart and soul of who we always were. At one point, a bumper crop of signs appeared on the walls describing a lofty hospital mission... compassion, respect, that sort of stuff... but I think most of the staff see a big disconnect between what the signs say and how things are really done. It's sad... I think we have lost sight of what we're all trying to do.

And

The energy in our hospital is incredible. I think that people have a real sense that what they do matters to our patients and to the community. We're not immune from hard times, but there's a level of trust that we're all in it together. The CEO does a lot to set the tone. He walks the walk... his office has a linoleum floor, he eats in the cafeteria and he knows your name. You know that if you have ideas or if you have concerns, somebody will listen. As a nurse, I have always worked hard, but I think I feel valued here more than any other place I've ever worked.

Here are two hospitals that may be similar in outward appearance... beds, facilities, staffing... but are vastly different in terms of organizational soul. I suspect there would not be much debate about where any of us would prefer to work, and I'd bet two more Red Sox tickets that the latter provides better (and more spiritually sensitive) patient care.

You can pick out a number of features that differentiate the two... the person and style of the CEO and the level of participation that employees feel, for instance. The particular feature that I am drawn to in these stories, however, is the very different experience of mission and purpose. The physician in the first story regretfully comments that the organization has *"lost sight of what we're all trying to do."* The nurse in the second description speaks about the sense that what they do *"matters to our patients and to the community."*

MISSION AND VALUES

Organizations with soul have a clear, meaningful, and shared sense of organizational purpose, and an understanding of the values that will enable them to realize that purpose.

I referred earlier to my 1996 sabbatical in Austin, Texas, working at a small spirituality center, the Seton Cove, affiliated with the Daughters of Charity Health Care System. Located in a former residence, the Cove was (and remains) a shaded and tranquil presence in the midst of a hot and bustling district where the parent medical center is located. It had been started several months prior to my arrival, being conceived as a place of hospitality and enriching conversation for leaders from the health care and business sectors of the community. With the visionary leadership of a dynamic 78-year-old Daughter of Charity, Sr. Mary Rose McPhee, the Cove focused particularly on the development of spiritual resources for these individuals and their organizations.

Throughout the medical center itself, there were aesthetically-appealing triptych panels on the walls describing organizational philosophy, mission and values. The centerpiece was the philosophy:

- *We serve each person as a Christian would serve Christ himself. As a caring community, we respect the dignity and needs of one another.*

A second panel defined the mission:

- *Our mission inspires us to care for and improve the health of those we serve with a special concern for the sick and the poor.*
- *We are called to be a sign of God's unconditional love for all and believe that all persons by their creation are endowed with dignity.*
- *Seton continues the Catholic tradition of service established by our founders: Vincent DePaul, Louise DeMarillac & Elizabeth Ann Seton.*

A third panel described the values: *The charity of Christ urges…*

- *Respect: A high regard for the worth of each person*
- *Quality service: Excellence in duty or work performed for others*
- *Simplicity: Honesty, integrity and straightforwardness.*
- *Advocacy for the poor: Supporting the cause of those who lack resources for a reasonable quality of life*
- *Inventiveness to infinity: Boundless creativity*

These statements do well in expressing Seton's core purpose and values. They also illustrate three reasons why a shared understanding of mission and values is important in organizations; providing energy, direction, and accountability.

Energy. A meaningful understanding of mission not only captures what the organization aspires to do; it creates energy by drawing attention to a purpose that can engage employees' hearts and passion. I recall Ken Melrose, the CEO of the Toro company, saying that employees didn't get particularly excited about making good lawn mowers, but did become engaged with the challenge of developing products that would serve the home care needs of customers in ways that were environmentally responsible and sustainable.

In the Seton statement of mission and values, one's attention is drawn to the centerpiece phrase, *as a Christian would serve Christ himself.* Abstract ideas like "respect" and "dignity" are meaningful as part of the Seton mission, but my reaction is that there is a much more profound level of reverence and sacredness with this centerpiece phrase, which I think engages the heart.

Similarly, in my exemplary practice research that I have described previously,[10] the *una voce* recitation by the community health center staffs that their mission was to "provide quality health care to people who otherwise would not have access to it" showed how powerful that purpose was in the work they did together.

Direction. The second feature of a shared understanding of mission and values is that it helps to chart the course of organizational decisions and directions. One can envision senior leaders in the Seton organization gathered around a conference table contemplating some decision about programs, financing, or staffing. Would it not help them to consider such questions as:

- How do *"special concern for the sick and the poor"* and *"supporting the cause of those who lack resources for a reasonable quality of life"* enter into this decision?

- What directions may be inspired by what we know of the lives of *Vincent DePaul, Louise DeMarillac & Elizabeth Ann Seton?* (You can perhaps picture a Seton version of the "WWJD; What Would Jesus Do?" bracelet: "WWVDPLDMEASD.")
- Might there be some choice that is relatively more consistent with *"honesty, integrity, and straightforwardness?"*

In my own organization, a part of our stated mission is to "Improve the health of Maine people, with particular emphasis on rural areas and underserved populations." There have been a number of conversations over the years that have turned on the questions of whether a particular choice "improved the health of Maine people," or perhaps particularly focused on the "rural and underserved people" in our communities. I recall a proposal from a behavioral health subcontractor, for instance, that would have provided individual services for private-pay patients and drop-in group services for uninsured patients. Enticing as it may have been to have additional behavioral health presence in our family practice centers, we decided as an organization that this proposal was not consistent with the mission of special regard for underserved people, and the proposal was declined.

Accountability. Third, a shared understanding of mission and values offers an approach to accountability. It can provide a template for evaluating organizational performance with respect to the processes and outcomes that the organizations have determined are most meaningful for them.

With a clear articulation of shared mission and values, the necessary organizational conversation about "How are we doing?" is grounded in the things that are organizationally "vital and sacred."

Conversations at the Seton Medical Center, for instance, might explore:

- *What does it mean for us to consider all persons as "endowed with dignity?"*

- *How are we doing in sustaining a culture of "respect?"*
- *What are the ways that we create a climate where employees feel empowered to be "boundlessly creative," and how can we nurture that?*

At the Maine-Dartmouth Family Medicine Residency, we have had lively and extraordinarily helpful conversations about our shared value of "Openness and appreciation of difference." Our organizational values were defined in a lengthy consensus process that I will describe shortly, and the idea of respecting and honoring the richness and diversity of human qualities and values in patients and staff has always been a fundamental tenet of our life together.

This value was not much tested in the early years. The program was founded in the early 1970s and initially attracted groups of resident physicians (as chronicled in John McPhee's classic essay, Heirs of General Practice[11]) who were predominantly white, Eastern-educated, progressive, back-to-the-earth types who had largely emigrated from privileged suburban backgrounds. In the early years, one heard the descriptors "granola" and "Birkenstock" regularly.

Gradually, things changed. For a variety of reasons, we began to attract a broader variety of resident physicians for training… individuals (good doctors all) who had more humble origins, who were politically and religiously more conservative, and many of whom came from international medical backgrounds. We wrestled… as we continue to wrestle… with what it means to welcome people from a diversity of backgrounds and to honor the variety and richness of experiences and beliefs that they bring. How can we be truly respectful to a red-state Republican in a political culture that is overwhelmingly blue? How can we accommodate and honor residents who are followers of Islam… or, for that matter, conservative Christians… in a residency community where these orientations stand out? What does it feel like in this organization for resident physicians from other countries… Iran, Iraq, China, Bosnia, Vietnam… who face the challenges of cultural isolation, learning medicine in a second language and dealing with very different assumptions about doctors, patients, and illness?

In the context of such differences, we have made a point to develop systems where we check in with one another about "How is it going?" with respect to this particular shared value. The definition of the value of "Openness and appreciation of difference," in other words, prompts us as a community to be accountable to revisiting how we are, in fact, making this a part of our organizational life.

DEVELOPING AN UNDERSTANDING OF MISSION AND VALUES

A shared understanding of mission and values comes from conversation. You will recall the observation by organizational consultant Margaret Wheatley, that "Real change begins with the simple act of people talking about what they care about[9]. "There is no power for change," she continues, "greater than a community discovering what it cares about." Soul grows in organizations in the power of people giving voice to their cherished values, visions, and hopes.

The conversation may take many forms.

- *"What are we doing here… what is our core purpose?"*
- *"How do we hope to create value for people coming through the door?"*
- *"What kind of community of people working together do we want to be?"*
- *"When are the times when we feel most alive and inspired doing our work together?*

Six suggestions about the process. First, the conversation about mission and values is a *positive* conversation, not a negative conversation. Identifying problems and institutional pathology can be helpful up to a point, but the vitality of the conversation flows from giving voice to where groups *want to be going* and how they may move there. The energy for change comes not from focusing on moving away from an undesired state, but from moving toward something that matters.

Most of us have been involved in conversations about team functioning when the conversation gravitated to a recitation of what was wrong. *"We need to do something about all the suspiciousness and back-stabbing." "We never know what anyone is doing around here... communication is really bad." "I feel like I am completely out of the loop in decision-making... I just hear about decisions getting handed down from somebody else."* It is important not to sweep emotions and issues under the rug, but the same principle holds for organizations as it does for clinical work; you have to turn the corner from a focus on what needs to change to the positively-framed conversations about where you want to go and how you are going to get there.

Second, this is an ***inclusive*** conversation. Mission is not defined by senior leaders in boardrooms. Everyone in the organization has some input, and some of the best ideas and most incisive observations often come from lower status staff members, in the same way that unvarnished truth often comes from peripheral participants in medical family meetings. I recall a receptionist saying how important it was to her that she could go to the practice manager and know that she would be listened to and respected, and I recall a medical assistant saying how much she cherished times when there was a little laughter and personal contact among staff, even on busy days. It is vitally important that observations such as these go into the hopper in developing an understanding of mission and values.

Third, ***stories*** often play a special and vital role in the conversation. Inviting people to recall and tell about times that have mattered to them in the life of the organization brings a spirit to the conversation that is more powerful than the same ideas expressed in conceptual form. One might ask:

- *When have been times when you have really felt like we are doing something meaningful here together?*

- *What are examples of times when we have been working together in ways that feel positive and affirming to you?*
- *What happens here that helps to draw out the best in people?*

Fourth, it is an ***iterative*** process. You solicit input. Somebody pulls people's perspectives about mission and values together into a draft statement. The draft is returned to stakeholders for their feedback. Somebody pulls together the feedback into a revised draft. This is returned to stakeholders for their feedback. The draft may be revised again and put out again for review. Successive iterations, in other words, are developed and reviewed until there is a consensus within the organization that you have it right.

Fifth, the process results in an articulation of mission and values that is ***concise and knowable.*** Laurie Beth Jones, author of a helpful book on personal understanding of mission, gives the example of a relative in the Korean War.[12] On sentry duty, he was trained to challenge approaching people with the command to identify themselves and "state your mission." If the approaching person was not able to respond to this within a few seconds, there was trouble.

Similarly, statements of mission and values… and, more broadly, the shared understanding of mission and values… need to be concise, knowable and engaging enough that staff carry them in their hearts. You might experiment with asking staff in your organization, "What is our mission?" or perhaps ask this of yourself. If staff don't know the answer, or if they have to flip over their ID to look at the statement of mission on the back, it is not clear enough, or not engaging enough, or both.

Sixth, the conversation about defining mission and values is not a static conversation; it is ***ongoing.*** The power of statements of mission comes not from precise one-time wordsmithing, but from the ongoing conversation about "how are we doing with the vision and values to which we have committed ourselves?" We will return to this idea.

I have referred a couple of times to the statement of mission and values from the Maine-Dartmouth Family Medicine Residency. This was developed over the course of about a year with the kind of inclusive and iterative process that I have described.

We began by defining the nature and breadth of the process and by telling some stories about sentinel events that had already taken place. The program had been founded with the express mission of providing quality health care to people with limited resources, who had previously received health care only inconsistently in a disconnected variety of clinics. As time went along, we took initiative in a number of areas, such as specifically recruiting women into Family Medicine, welcoming osteopathic physicians at a time when they were not generally accepted in allopathic circles, and starting the first family-centered birthing room process in the region. We had always been a fairly non-hierarchical organization, where interns addressed the director as "Alex" and immediately had a full-share voice in how policies were developed. We had always emphasized community medicine, and many residents and faculty had been involved in the legislative process in the workings of state government, with the state capital being about as far away as a fly ball to the warning track.

Growing out of this collection of stories about the kind of organization we had been, we invited input about the mission and values that should guide us, going forward. We staged interviews and some group conversations with all of the constituencies who were involved with the residency… faculty, residents, medical students, board members, graduates, hospital administration, clinical and administrative staff, support staff, and patients. We developed summaries of conversations and draft statements of mission and values that were reviewed and revised several times. In the end, we had a consensus articulation of what is "vital and sacred" for our organization:

- Mission
  - Educate physicians for a lifetime of competent, compassionate and personally satisfying practice.
  - Improve the health of Maine people, with particular emphasis on rural areas and underserved populations.

- o Promote the involvement of physicians in the life of the broader community.
- Residency Values
  - o Creating a community of learners which...
    - ▪ Honors our patient care responsibilities.
    - ▪ Balances learning and patient care in a way that combines scientific rigor and humanity.
    - ▪ Values the contributions of other community caregivers.
  - o Creating a workplace culture that fosters...
    - ▪ Respect and teamwork.
    - ▪ Support for personal well-being.
    - ▪ Openness and appreciation of difference.

STRATEGY 19
Talk about the mission

Begin... or renew... a conversation in your organization about mission and values. I have suggested a number of conversation-starters in this chapter, and surely you can come up with your own, as well.

If you have an organizational statement of mission and values, sit down with a colleague and talk about it. How well does it capture the values that move people in the organization? How are you doing with respect to the values that this statement articulates? How could you do better? Why is this conversation important?

If your organization does not have a statement of mission and values, reflect with your colleague about what a statement would say if you did have one. What words would capture the values that you aspire to, at your best, as an organization? Why does this conversation matter? How might it enhance the vitality and focus of the organization if you had a wider conversation? How, indeed, could you have a wider conversation?

MISSION AND VALUES AS PART
OF ORGANIZATIONAL LIFE

Articulating an understanding of mission and core values is an important process for health care organizations, but it can't end there. The reason to engage this process, after all, is to create the kind of organizational culture or "soul" that will be affirming and empowering for staff and healing for patients. The conversation about mission and values, therefore, has to be an active and ongoing part of organizational life. There are a number of places to engage this conversation.

Recruitment of new employees. Prospective interns who are considering applying to our program are mailed a chunky packet about the program with a statement of mission and values on top… the first page of information about us that they see. The statement of mission and values also occupies a prominent location on the residency Internet home page, www.mainedartmouth.org. In any health care organization, communicating mission and values to prospective employees helps them to decide whether they might wish to work there, and begins a process of orientation to the culture if they end up doing so.

Orientation of new employees. The director of a homeless shelter describes:

> Bud was a quiet guy, mostly. We knew he had had a rough life but he never said much about himself. He'd make a little money, rent a room for a while, then he would blow it all in a bar and be back on the streets… and end up here. When he was sober, he was just a polite, quiet and frail guy in the background. When he was drunk, he could get foul-mouthed and abusive. He never hit anybody here… rumor had it he had done some hard time earlier in his life… but we had to ask him to leave more than a few times. He passed on a couple of years ago. I remember a few weeks before he died, he was here for the last time and called me aside. I'll never forget… he said he knew he had been a "pain in the ass" a lot,

but he wanted me to know that in his whole life, this was the one place where he had really felt welcome, and he wanted me to know how much that meant to him. I was touched, and I make a point of telling this story to all our staff as they come on board because that says better than I could the kind of place we try to be.

Orientation can be an engaging time to introduce new staff to organizational culture and values, and stories can be a particularly engaging way to approach it. Our own orientation of new residents has often included a presentation of some "oral history" from a senior faculty member of some sentinel events in the life of our organization. Through this story-telling and conversation about our mission and values, we want to introduce new employees to the qualities of organizational culture that have sustained the program for over forty years, and for which they will become the current generation of stewards.

Retreats. A nurse recounts:

We have done well over the years having one or two off-site retreats a year, for the leadership team and for the whole group. We tried having various outside people leading it... we've had motivational speakers and people from HR... but the best times have been when we just spend time with each other and talk about the hard times and especially the joys that hold us together.

Off-site retreats can be a particularly good time for the "How are we doing?" conversation. A few hours free of daily clinical and administrative responsibilities can provide a rich opportunity to review the organization's mission and value commitments, affirming people's positive efforts and exploring together what could happen to realize the organization's values even more fully.

A dynamic model for staging this conversation is Appreciative Inquiry. Developed by David L. Cooperrider and Ronald Fry at the Case Weatherhead School of Management, the AI perspective searches for what is best in organizations... for an understanding of what happens that enable organizations to be most successful, creative, and alive. Analogous to our conversation about the clinical emphasis of moving toward solutions rather than away from problems, AI emphasizes the identification and nurturing of positive and hopeful times, rather than defining and somehow moving away from organizational problems. Points of conversation, therefore, might be:

- *When is our work together most effective and how does that happen?*
- *When are the times when we best give expression to our shared value of "openness and appreciation of difference?"*
- *What is it that we can most take pride in over the last few months?*
- *What is it that keeps us coming to work here?*

The Appreciative Inquiry "Commons," http://appreciative-inquiry.case.edu/, offers background, essays, extensive research, and manuals and practical tools.

Celebrations. Gathering for celebrations can provide opportunities for health care staff to look with fondness and pride at what they have been doing together. Celebrations that recognize service anniversaries, retirements, or colleagues moving to other positions tend to be times when there is some reflective talk about things that matter.

As an educational program, we follow an annual cycle of academic life, with new interns arriving and senior residents completing their training in the second half of June. For many years, we have had an annual graduation observance to celebrate the contributions of our departing residents and to wish them well as they launch into practice as physicians. We recognize our graduating residents with a healthy dose of roasting, with outrageous skits that incisively point to their foibles (along with those of the faculty) and with some words of earnest tribute that point to the particular gifts and goodness that these young men and women bring to medicine.

Inevitably, the conversation and recognition call forth the values that bind us together as an organization... caring for underserved people, being engaged in the community, honoring patient care responsibilities, respect, and teamwork. I don't recall anyone ever specifically quoting the mission statement, but one certainly leaves this occasion with a refreshed and reinvigorated view of the mission and values in which we all join.

There are, of course, no end of approaches to energizing the role of mission and values in the life of health care organizations. Other organizations have worked with such venues as annual reviews and check-ins, mentoring programs, employee forums, reflection questions, formative reading, and renewal days for staff.[13, 14]

I should also mention an intriguing practice in the Roman Catholic tradition, the Vice President for Mission Effectiveness. Catholic health care organizations typically have a person with this title appointed at the senior leadership level, whose role it is to oversee the incorporation of mission values in organizational life. I suspect that the impact of this position varies somewhat with the person who serves in this role and with the leadership culture of the organization, but at its best, it is an opportunity for one person to champion the awareness and honoring of shared values.

STRATEGY 20
Keep talking and develop a
wider view of mission and values

You have now invited a colleague for some good coffee and begun the conversation about mission and values. Building on this foundation, explore ways to expand the conversation. Perhaps you can advocate for developing an organized, shared understanding of mission and values if your organization does not have one. Perhaps you can bring a reminder and consideration about mission and values into discussions of what your organization is doing, and why. Perhaps you can talk among a wider group of people about the places where you can best bring the energy and spirit of the things that matter to you into the life of your organization.

ORGANIZATIONAL SPECIALISTS

What, no reference to organizational assessment paradigms? Aren't there instruments out there for evaluating the culture of organizations? What about the 31 Keys to Organizational Vitality?

The answers are: "Correct," "Yes," and "No such thing," respectively. There are indeed a prodigious collection of resource materials available for organizational assessment and for theories and models of organizational change. You will see at your local bookseller that the "Management" and "Business" sections occupy as much shelf space as the great works of world literature.

Much of the application of this knowledge, however, falls in the purview of organizational specialists. People go to business schools to learn these things. People get degrees in organizational psychology to learn these things. People are employed as organizational development specialists, human resources directors, and consultants.

The more specialized approaches in the organizational world, in other words, fall to specialists… in the same way that the more specialized approaches to spiritual diagnosis and spiritual suffering fall to specialist spiritual caregivers. For the rest of us who are not organizational specialists, the point that I want to emphasize is earnest conversation, with an open heart. One does not need an organizational diagnosis paradigm in order to initiate an earnest conversation with somebody else about what you care about.

SUMMARY

- Organizations have souls. Cultivating the soul of health care organizations empowers staff to provide good spiritual care and creates welcoming and healing environments that are themselves vital aspects of good spiritual care.
- There are data that qualities of organizational soul… per-

taining to mission, community, and leadership… make a difference with measures of staff well-being, patient satisfaction, and with process and health care outcome variables.

- A shared understanding of organizational mission and values provides energy, direction, and accountability.
- A shared understanding of organizational mission and values is created in conversation… as Margaret Wheatley says, "a community discovering what it cares about."
- Principles for the conversation about organizational mission and values include:
  o It is a positive conversation.
  o It is an inclusive conversation.
  o Stories play a vital role in the conversation.
  o It is an iterative process.
  o Well-framed statements of mission and values are concise and knowable.
  o The conversation about mission and values is not static; it is ongoing.
- Places to engage conversations about mission and values include:
  o Recruitment of new employees
  o Orientation of new employees
  o Retreats
  o Celebrations
- Organizational specialists can offer more specific and targeted approaches. For the rest of us, the key is earnest conversation with an open heart.

REFERENCES

1. Bolman LG, Deal TE. *Leading with Soul: An Uncommon Journey of Spirit*. San Francisco: Jossey-Bass; 2001.
2. Briskin A. *The Stirring of Soul in the Workplace*. San Francisco: Berrett-Koehler; 1998.
3. Chappell T. *The Soul of a Business*. New York: Bantam; 1993.

4. Conger JA, ed. *Spirit at Work: Discovering the Spirituality in Leadership*. San Francisco: Jossey-Bass; 1994.

5. Gallagher RS. *The Soul of an Organization*: Dearborn; 2003.

6. Mitroff II, Denton EA. *A Spiritual Audit of Corporate America: A Hard Look at Spirituality, Religion, and Values in the Workplace*. San Francisco: Jossey-Bass; 1999.

7. Owen H. *The Power of Spirit: How Organizations Transform*. San Francisco: Berrett-Koehler; 2000.

8. Toms M, ed. *The Soul of Business*. Carlsbad, CA: New Dimensions Foundation; 1997.

9. Wheatley M. *Turning to One Another: Simple Conversations to Restore Hope to the Future*. San Francisco: Berrett-Koehler; 2002.

10. Craigie FC, Jr., Hobbs RF. Exploring the organizational culture of exemplary community health center practices. *Fam Med.* 2004;36(10):733-738.

11. McPhee J. *Heirs of General Practice*. New York: Farrar, Straus and Giroux; 1986.

12. Jones L. *The Path: Creating Your Mission Statement for Work and for Life*. New York: Hyperion; 1998.

13. Richardt SS, et al. *Spirituality and Spiritual Formation*. Evansville, IN: Daughters of Charity National Health System - East Central Region; 1995.

14. Craigie FC, Jr. Weaving spirituality into organizational life. Suggestions for processes and programs. *Health Prog.* Mar-Apr 1998;79(2):25-28, 32.

Chapter Twelve

Cultivate Community

*Reclaiming soul in health care must address a deep human need
for community and friendships. We social creatures need each other
not only for company but also for meaning in our lives.*[1]

Linda G. Henry and James D. Henry

A patient registrar reflects,

*We're like a family here. It's not so much that we get together outside
of work... sometimes we do, but not really often... but there's a lot of
day to day caring. People notice how you're doing, and somebody puts
a hand on your shoulder if you're having a hard time. When you get
overwhelmed, somebody appears to pitch in. When my mom was dying
a couple of years ago, some of my friends here donated vacation days so
I could spend more time with her... and most of the staff, including the
providers, went to the funeral. When my son's basketball team went to
the state finals, everybody wore some green and white, the school colors.
Sometimes I think I'd come to work here to be with my work family
even if they didn't pay me.*

Organizations with soul have a strong spirit of community. As
this registrar suggests, colleagues in spirited organizations may or

may not be best friends outside of work, but there is a clear sense of caring and commitment to one another… like a supportive family… in the workplace.

This spirit of community matters. It is a vital part of spiritual care. A primary care nurse comments,

We have a good sense of community here. We care about each other. It's a contagious atmosphere… if somebody is kind or encouraging to you, you feel good and you pass it along to somebody else. We know that we have a serious job to do, but you have to make it as positive and enjoyable as you can.

She continues,

I think the atmosphere here is really important for patients, too. They pick up on it pretty quickly. If there was a lot of bickering and complaining, then patients… who often don't feel good anyway… wouldn't want to be here. If they see us being happy and helping each other out, they feel good and welcome in coming here, and I really believe that they'll get better care… because it's clear to me that more satisfied people provide better patient care.

In the last chapter, we considered ways in which the shared understanding of organizational mission and values can energize groups of people working together. We turn our attention now to qualities of community in health care organizations, and how they may similarly help to create the kind of caring, affirming, and healing environments that the registrar and nurse are speaking about.

COMMUNITY IN HEATH
CARE ORGANIZATIONS

When I last visited my local bookseller, steel rule in hand, I found that there were 14 feet, 6 ¾ inches of accumulated wisdom about culture in organizational life. Management, leadership (which we will explore further in the next chapter), motivational techniques, and approaches guaranteed to result in successful and productive organizations… it can feel overwhelming.

It occurs to me that the process of molding organizational culture bears some similarity to our conversation about spirituality itself. I have suggested that it is less important that you buy into my definition of spirituality and my specific approaches than it is that you filter through the ideas that we are considering and develop approaches for defining and working with spirituality that feel right for you. How you speak with a 69 year old man with advanced liver disease will be different from how I would speak with that man, and it is more important that you be true to your own style and your own heart than it is that you be true to mine.

So, too, with organizational culture and forming community in your own workplace. The challenge is not to become facile with the whole 14 ½ feet, but to look at some key ideas, bring to bear your own wisdom and experience, and identify some approaches that feel right for you.

In that spirit, I want to describe some of the ways that I have come to think about cultivating community in health care organizations. These ideas come both from my long tenure and periodic consulting in health care organizations and from empirical data, particularly from exemplary practice research.

Exemplary practice research offers a rich source of ideas about the factors that help organizations to function at their best. Perhaps the most remarkable example of this type of research comes from Dartmouth Medical School, where a large group of investigators from the worlds of clinical medicine and public health conducted studies on exemplary clinical "microsystems" in the early years of this decade.[2,3] They developed a detailed and multi-layered process of nominations and validation of highly performing clinical "microsystems" across the United States… small, front-line units of clinical care. They identified 20 such exemplary clinical microsystems across a range of medical practice specialties and engaged a multi-factorial qualitative and quantitative research methodology to explore the central question of what makes these programs so good.

My own research, to which I have referred before, has looked at exemplary community health centers in Maine.[4] Using a similar (albeit more humble) process of nominations and validation in a state-wide search of primary care practices, I identified two high-performing community health centers that, practically speaking, were considered to be great places to work and great places to be a patient. With my colleague Rick Hobbs, MD, I then used a qualitative methodology... extracting data from interviews and field observation... to develop themes about the same question; "What makes these places so good?"

POSITIVE QUALITIES OF COMMUNITY IN HEALTH CARE ORGANIZATIONS

Arising out of this personal and research body of experience, I see two aspects of community in health care organizations. There are aspects of community that have to do with the "business" of people working together... collaboration and teamwork... and aspects of community having to do with the more personal and affective relationships of people working together.

Collaboration and teamwork

In health care organizations with soul, staff invest energy and heart in the business of working together. This takes various forms.

Sharing the workload. Staff are attentive to the workload of their colleagues and make efforts to help out in ways that go beyond their particular job descriptions. A practice manager describes:

Everybody pitches in and helps when they see that somebody needs it. If someone has a little slack time and someone else is really busy, they'll just slide in and help out. If you can do it, you do. If I walk by and the front desk is swamped and the phone is ringing, I'll pick up the phone and do the phone for a few minutes. If the records clerks are swamped, people go in there and help with charts. This has always been a place where people help each other out and it really feels good to know that you have that kind of caring and support from your co-workers.

A physician comments,

We put a lot of emphasis here on creating giving relationships, rather than demanding or adversarial relationships. If we can genuinely try to help each other out, even though sometimes it's not convenient, it's just a much healthier relationship and people are willing to give and bend a little as opposed to trying to protect their own turf. If it's a relationship of "You do your thing and I'll do my thing and I'm not going to help you out," then you create a polarized atmosphere that becomes adversarial and doesn't work. The whole attitude is that it's going to be a cooperative relationship… we have a job to do and how can we do it best as a team and share the load.

Everybody counts. It is clearly understood and demonstrated, in the culture of these organizations, that everyone is valued for their contributions and for their opinions. From a records clerk:

Every person is valued as a team member. It doesn't matter where you work in this building… each person's thoughts are valued. I can't help out much in a conversation about Medicare reimbursement… Part A and Part B and all that stuff… but I think I can contribute some pretty good ideas about the work flow and how patients move through the system, and I've found that people really listen. I can go to [practice manager] and suggest something and she'll really listen respectfully and think it through with me and help to move the idea along if she thinks it's good. Some other places I've worked, I'm just "the woman with the GED" around a bunch of people with all these degrees and I usually haven't gotten the time of day. It feels so much better here, and it makes you want to be involved in making things as good as possible.

From a medical assistant:

We all work as a team here. Everybody counts, no matter what your title is. People don't feel uncomfortable asking because "she's a file clerk" and "he's a doctor."

Safety and affirmation. Staff in these organizations feel affirmed and safe in doing their jobs and being creative in the workplace. Motivation is from shared purpose and commitment, not fear. A receptionist describes:

It's easier to be yourself here, to relax here. You can do what you have to do without being afraid you're going to mess up and someone's going to get mad at you. Everybody is laid back and they're very understanding. Where I've worked before, people take more pleasure in telling you what you're doing wrong than what you're doing right.

A physician assistant comments,

Part of what makes the atmosphere here great is that people respect each other. You can feel free to open up in the staff meetings, knowing that people will listen and you will not be judged.

Dealing with conflict and moving on. Soulful health care organizations are not immune from conflict, but they look squarely at the issues that present, work them through, and move on. From a laboratory technician:

We have the same stresses that other places do, but people say what they need to say and move on. They don't dwell on things or keep them buried or stew on them.

From a nurse:

When a problem comes up, we deal with the problem. We don't go off on tangents about people's personalities. The person is not the problem; the problem is what has to be dealt with. We really work together to understand why problems are happening and what we can do to make situations better. Nobody gets attacked, and everybody is included in the problem-solving. Rather than saying "you're the problem," we work together to look for solutions.

I might add that soulful health care organizations are not particularly slow-paced and relaxed environments in terms of workload. To the contrary, the community health centers that I examined… and this seems to be the case with the clinical microsystems in the Dartmouth research, as well… are fairly high-volume, fast-paced practices. The key issue with organizational soul, in other words, is clearly not the amount of work that these organizations do; it is the ways in which staff collaborate in the work that they do.

From a medical assistant:

We all keep running until the work is done. You can see that we're stressed in the way we walk or the expressions on our faces, but we never let it get out of control and we don't let it take over the way we try to work with each other.

Another physician comments,

Work is difficult and stressful, but the overriding spirit is one of friendliness and joy.

Personal and affective aspects of community

Not only do people work collaboratively in soulful organizations: they care about each other. It may be that this, in fact, comes first… that a personal commitment of colleagues to care about and respect one another underlies the kinds of collaboration that we have just considered. Personal engagement among staff also takes several forms.

Knowing and caring. People in these exemplary practices tend, simply, to enjoy each other. They know one another and care about one another. A practice manager comments,

People here vary in how private they are, but I think we're all sen-

sitive to what is happening with each other and we try to support our colleagues in the hard times and to celebrate with them in the good times. When my granddaughter was born, several of the staff took me out to lunch. When [social worker's] husband was dying of cancer, we tried really hard to give her space and also to be there for her when she just needed to talk to somebody. We had a little party last week for one of our medical assistants who just finished phlebotomy training and will be moving over to the hospital. People are always passing around photographs of their kids and their pets and their vacation trips. Nobody has to be any more public about their personal lives than they're comfortable being, but I think that all of the staff are genuinely interested in each other as people. It really makes a difference to work in a place where people care who you are.

Along the same lines, I recall a conversation a number of years ago with a nurse educator who had been doing research about inpatient medical units. In a large metropolitan medical center, she used a variation of an exemplary practice methodology to identify units of care that were functioning well and those that were functioning less well. Within the medical center complex, all of the units had similar layouts that included a large bulletin board between the nursing stations and break rooms. She found that these bulletin boards, on the well-functioning units, were covered with family photos, community announcements, humorous cartoons, and the like. The bulletin boards on the less well functioning units tended to be covered with tidy, carefully-aligned statements of policies and procedures.

Day to day attentiveness and support. In these soulful organizations, the commitment of knowing and caring about one another is played out both in the larger events of life… like graduations and serious illnesses… and in the smaller expressions of support in day-to-day workplace life. You read the example, at the beginning of this chapter, of the patient registrar commenting that "people notice how you're doing, and somebody puts a hand on your shoulder if you're having a hard time."

A triage nurse, similarly, says

We all have things that come up on our personal lives, or just things here at work, and if we share that with somebody else, they're always willing to listen. If somebody is tense, somebody else will see it and do something to relax that person... a joke, a neck rub, a listening ear.

A physician describes:

One of our medical assistants had a son who was in New York on 9/11. As we all became aware of that, another medical assistant who had been on vacation that day volunteered to come in and take over for her so that she could go home and try to get in touch with her son. I was so touched by that... there was no sense of duty or obligation, just one person being kind and generous to another person that she cared about.

Laughter and fun. Finally, these organizations are not serious and grimly resolute in performing their work; there is, as the physician commented above, a "spirit... of joy." A billing clerk says,

We take our work seriously, but we don't take ourselves too seriously.

A physician assistant adds,

Things can get so hectic around, here, you have to sit back and laugh at yourself. We get foolish at times, and humor helps us to get through it and makes it doable, rather than screaming or crying.

And from a social worker:

We come to work for serious reasons... providing good health care to people... but we also come to work because we enjoy the people we work with. We joke around a lot, during the day when you can and always at staff meetings. Someone will come in with a funny story or

something that made them laugh. And we always have food... no one is anorectic around here.

STRATEGY 21
Define positive qualities of workplace community

You now have my delineation of some qualities of soulful workplace environments from my observations and research. What resonates with you? How would you put into words the qualities of community in the workplace that matter to you? The types of reflective questions that I suggest are, by now, familiar to you:

- What do you see happening in the workplace that enlivens you and your colleagues, and brings out your best?
- When have been times when you really felt a genuine spirit of collaboration and caring among the people you work with?
- In addition to the clinical mission that you perform, what keeps you coming to work in terms of the relationships you have with your colleagues?
- What have you been able to do... and what can you do... to contribute to a spirit of collaboration and caring in your organization?

CULTIVATING COMMUNITY

In Chapter 11, we considered a number of places to engage conversations about mission and values in organizations; recruitment of new employees, orientation of new employees, retreats, and celebrations. These settings are certainly well suited to cultivating community, as well; they provide opportunities both to *talk about* community and to *practice* community.

I make a practice of getting to know colleagues in my organization. Some are more or less accessible than others, but I make a point of following my natural curiosity about what people take pride in, what they enjoy, what they do for fun, where they live, how they came to Maine, who is in their families, and other such questions that help me to know the people behind the roles.

Remarkable stories, all. The colleague down the hall who was in the Peace Corps and moonlights doing energy audits. The resident who has professionally played upright bass. The medical assistant who does exquisite stained glass, and another who owns a horse and spends summer weekends harness racing. The student who was the first person in her extended family to go to college. The Islamic colleague who just purchased a small building with several other people of his religious community that they will use for Friday prayers. The mild-mannered, soft-spoken graphic designer who puts my spirituality symposium brochure together who does gigs on weekends as the lead singer of the band, *Susie and the Smelts*. (Only in Maine!) The administrative assistant who is a kind and generous person whose life centers around her children whom she adores. It certainly heightens my appreciation in being a part of this organization to know these and so many other people a little better, and I hope that my knowing them and being known to them heightens their appreciation of being a part of this organization, as well.

I want to highlight five particular approaches to cultivating community in health care organizations.

Let go of the imperfections. One of the classic resources on community comes from German theologian Dietrich Bonhoeffer. In the couple of years before his death at the hands of the Nazis in 1945, Bonhoeffer had been involved in an underground seminary and wrote about his experiences of fellowship there in a short book called "Life Together."[5] Bonhoeffer argues that even among people who come together with religious intention, community will always have imperfections. It is destructive, he continues, for people to hold onto the "wish dream" of community being something that it cannot be. Conversely, it is the first step in creating genuine community when a group of people can let go of the ideal of perfection and be thankful for the simple fact of journeying together.

While we don't necessarily hold our health care organizations up to the same holy standards of Bonhoeffer's seminary, the principle is still relevant. We may care about the spirit of community in our practices and we may invest energy and heart in cultivating community, but it will always end up being short of perfection. As the receptionist who was speaking about the practice climate of safety suggested, there is a cost associated with being too vigilant and engaged with what is wrong in community life, and it is more empowering for people to be "laid back and understanding" about imperfection, in the service of moving together toward goals that matter to everyone.

Be the change. Famously, Gandhi is quoted as teaching that we need to "be the change that you wish to see in the world." So it is with cultivating a spirit of soulful community in health care organizations.

Whatever your responses are to Exercise 21, be that change. Do you value the "knowing and caring" in workplace relationships? Take the initiative to know and care. Is it important to you to have a workplace culture that feels safe for individual initiative and creativity? Extend a spirit of openness to others' initiatives. Do you value teamwork and collaboration? Look for ways to draw in your colleagues on projects that you can pursue together.

Tell stories. As you have heard me say several times, stories have more power than concepts. Stories highlight and give life to aspects of community relationships in ways that conceptual descriptions do not.

It is one thing to say that a chief resident is a good leader. It is something else to describe:

This last rotation, she was organized and she held other residents accountable and she was really supportive. I think she set a good tone for morning report, being clear about resident colleagues needing to be on time and to give succinct and focused presentations. Several days, she brought in articles for the group to review about patients… like that young girl with the acetaminophen overdose in the ICU. And I was really impressed the way she took [intern colleague] aside when he was devastated about the stillborn delivery and supported him making his way through it.

Make staff meetings open and empowering. I have seen a number of health care organizations where attending staff meetings wasn't necessarily a fate worse than death, but perhaps a fate on a par with dismemberment or incapacitation. You have seen this, too; meetings that the powerful people consistently avoid and the lower-level staff members begrudgingly attend because they have to.

Not so with the best-practice community health centers. Consider:

Our staff meetings help us to keep everything together. Each person is addressed, each person has a chance to speak, each person is validated. I know of staff meetings at other places where one person directs it and says "this is the way it will be." Amen, end of story. That's not the way it is here.

We have been adamant over the years in keeping our weekly staff meeting. We have often been asked to cut back, to use that time to see more patients, but we have stuck to our guns… it is such a big part of keeping everybody together. The staff meeting is the place where we get to unload. If somebody has a problem, we all get to find out about it and work together on how we can change things and make it better. Like last week, when the transcriptionist had some problems with the providers and she brought them some information about what was happening and asked if they could help her to make it better. It's wonderful that the providers will take the time to sit down with the staff like this.

The culture in this practice is that everybody works together, and that every person is as important as another. One big way the providers reinforce this is by being invested in staff meetings. They don't have a provider meeting and a nursing meeting, and all these different meetings... they have staff meetings where any member of the team can speak up about an issue and work through a problem. If there's a system broken, they involve everybody in fixing it. I know that in a lot of other practices, the providers don't like staff meetings... they don't understand why they have to be in a meeting with the receptionists. They see meetings with the whole staff as a waste of time. That's not the culture here.

A lot of solutions to issues get worked out at staff meeting. If someone feels like their job has grown too large as the practice has grown, for instance, we'll put their responsibilities on a flip chart and do some prioritizing together and see what we could do differently.

Clearly, the staff meetings in these exemplary practices bring people together, help them to feel valued, and provide settings for productive collaboration on issues and processes that affect the way they work.

The how-are-we-doing-here conversation (revisited). The fifth approach to cultivating community revisits the conversation about how things are going. With other people in your organization, you explore such questions as:

- *What are the features of our relationships with one another that are most important to us, and how are we doing?*
- *When are times when we see the best in one another, and how do these times come about?*
- *When have we been surprised or touched by some expression of goodness in our relationships together?*
- *What has happened here in the last month that we value and we would like to see continue?*
- *How could we move closer to becoming more consistently the kind of community we wish to be?*

STRATEGY 22
Choose some next steps in building goodness in your workplace community, and bring a colleague into the conversation

You have suggestions from me about approaches to cultivating positive workplace community and you have, of course, your own experience and wisdom as well. Growing out of these ideas, choose one or two approaches you can pursue that may stand to bring some additional goodness and good spirit to your working group. Brew up some more fair trade coffee and have an earnest conversation with a colleague about your thoughts and initiatives and invite their own reactions and wisdom.

SUMMARY

- Cultivating the soul of health care organizations empowers staff to provide good spiritual care and creates welcoming and healing environments that are themselves vital aspects of good spiritual care.
- Organizations with soul have a strong sense of community.
- Spirited health care organizations with a strong sense of community have characteristic features of collaboration and teamwork.
  - o Sharing the workload
  - o Everybody counts
  - o Safety and affirmation
  - o Dealing with conflict and moving on
- Spirited health care organizations also have characteristic features of personal and affective aspects of community.
  - o Knowing and caring
  - o Day to day attentiveness and support
  - o Laughter and fun
- Approaches to cultivating positive community in health care organizations include:

- ○ Letting go of imperfections
- ○ Being the change
- ○ Telling stories
- ○ Making staff meetings open and empowering
- ○ Revisiting the how-are-we-doing-here conversation

REFERENCES

1. Henry LG, Henry JD. *Reclaiming Soul in Health Care*. Chicago: Health Forum; 1999.
2. Nelson EC, Batalden PB, Huber TP, et al. Microsystems in health care: Part 1. Learning from high-performing front-line clinical units. *Jt Comm J Qual Improv.* Sep 2002;28(9):472-493.
3. Huber TP, Godfrey MM, Nelson EC, Mohr JJ, Campbell C, Batalden PB. Microsystems in health care: Part 8: Developing people and improving work life: What front-line staff told us. *Joint Commission Journal on Quality and Safety.* 2003;29(10):512-522.
4. Craigie FC, Jr., Hobbs RF. Exploring the organizational culture of exemplary community health center practices. *Fam Med.* 2004;36(10):733-738.
5. Bonhoeffer D. *Life Together: The Classic Exploration of Faith in Community*. San Francisco, CA: HarperSanFrancisco; 1976.

## Chapter Thirteen

Exercise Empowering Leadership

Outstanding business leaders understand that you really can't get people
to do things; you can only encourage them to want to do things.
And this encouragement is not through fear,
but through meaning, love, and hope. [1]

Richard McKnight, PhD

A family physician recounts,

One of the concrete things I feel best about over the years is starting
a birthing room at our hospital. This was at a time when the medical
consciousness was that childbirth was really a surgical event, and women
were whisked off from regular patient rooms to an operating room as it
was clear that they were about to deliver. I remember looking around
after one delivery at all the medical paraphernalia and thinking that
it was really sad, at least for normal deliveries... really sterile and
impersonal. Why couldn't we make labor and delivery a more peaceful
experience, and have children born into the world in a home-like en-
vironment, rather than a clinical one?

The more I thought about it, the more excited I got. It just seemed
natural. So I just started talking about it. First it was the people I knew
well and knew would be able to be supportive and creative with me.

Then I got together more people in a wider circle... the head nurse on OB, an administrator who was pretty open-minded, the hospital volunteer coordinator. I wanted to have a group of people whose opinions I thought would be helpful and who would either be involved with a decision about changing what we did or would be taken seriously by people higher up who would be making that decision.

We kicked around ideas... that were really novel at the time... about having one comfortable suite for labor and delivery, with regular furniture, a refrigerator, music, incandescent lights, homey decorations, and so forth. I was eager but I knew I needed to be patient. I did a lot of listening... people had questions about issues of cleanliness, liability, control, emergencies... and we hashed out the significance of these concerns and how we might work with them. I wanted us all to come back to the core question of what would be best for women and families... things that would make it a really peaceful and comforting experience for women and families. The more we kept talking, focusing on that, it was gratifying to see the way more and more people signed on and really contributed some good ideas of their own.

In the end, we put together a proposal that fairly covered the concerns that people raised and came with enough credibility that the administration was willing to give it a shot. Of course, it turned out to be spectacularly successful and it's really the expectation these days.

A nice example of practical, informal leadership. It shows a number of signs of spirited leadership in health care, to which we will return:

- *"...the more excited I got"*
- *"...just started talking."*
- *"...got together more people in a wider circle"*
- *"...needed to be patient."*
- *"...did a lot of listening..."*
- *"...hashed out... these concerns..."*
- *"...wanted us all to come back to the core question"*
- *"...people... contributed some good ideas of their own."*

LEADERSHIP AND SPIRITUAL CARE

In several preceding chapters, we have examined the premise that the spirit, or "soul," of health care organizations reflects a vital dimension of spiritual care. Along with the "personal" and the "clinical" arenas of spiritual care, the organizational arena is important because soulful organizations are spiritually empowering for staff, and welcoming and healing for patients.

Soulful organizations, in turn, are energized and directed by a shared understanding of mission and values (Chapter 11), and are sustained by a community spirit of collaboration and caring (Chapter 12).

In this context, positive health care leadership is essential in providing good spiritual care for three reasons.

Good leadership is good for clinicians

Meaning is good for the soul. You will recall our definition of spiritual care: "helping people to connect with the things that really matter to them." Finding meaning by connecting with the core things that really matter… relationships, community activities, social causes, workplace directions… is enlivening in general, and sustaining and healing in adversity.

Giving expression to the best that is within us is also good for the soul. The Positive Psychology data and literature that we have reviewed suggest that emotional and spiritual well-being is associated with giving expression to the personal qualities and strengths that are personally most important to us. If I am hard-wired to be passionate about creativity… or justice… or compassion… or hope… and find ways to give expression to those qualities, I am likely to experience satisfaction and joy to an extent that I would otherwise not have experienced.

Leadership provides opportunities for both… for personal meaning and for the expression of personally important qualities of character. Simply put, taking the initiative to exercise health care leadership is good for the soul.

I walked away from the meeting where I volunteered to serve on the task force looking at nursing staff reorganization and wondered what in the world I had done. I was probably ten years to thirty years younger than everybody else and I'd been out of nursing school myself only three or four years. What could I possibly contribute? Over the next few days, I think I realized that this was really important to me because it had to do with the professional satisfaction and, really, the future of my profession... at least, here at this hospital. So, if anything, I had more at stake as a younger person than my senior colleagues. It occurred to me that it would have been easier not to have gotten involved, but that I really had to get involved because this was where my heart... my soul... was leading me.

Good leadership is good for staff

Good health care leadership empowers staff. In one of the landmark business books of the last two decades, Edgar Schein argued that the principal role of leaders is the development and nurturing of corporate culture.[2] Leadership that moves and sustains organizational culture in the directions that we described from exemplary practice research... sharing the workload, everybody counts, safety and affirmation, dealing with conflict and moving on, knowing and caring, day to day attentiveness and support, and laughter and fun... helps staff to be engaged in their work and supportive of one another.

Good leadership is good for patients

Of course, patients benefit when good leadership results in concrete, positive changes in health care systems. The birthing experience will be richer for women and families at the hospital where the physician in the story beginning this chapter practices.

Patients also benefit by means of Reasons #1 and #2. Exercising leadership is good for the soul, and spiritually-grounded clinicians provide better spiritual care. Good leadership forms good organizational culture, and soulful organizations provide better spiritual care, as well.

WINDOWS ON HEALTH CARE LEADERSHIP: VOICES OF CLINICIANS

Along with culture in organizational life, leadership is a hot topic at your local bookseller. Leadership is elucidated by management gurus, visionary CEOs, legendary sports coaches, failed office-seekers, medieval mystics, generals (living and dead), and Jesus Himself. Amid this flurry of writing, there is strikingly little commentary on leadership provided by health care clinicians.

I am especially intrigued by what clinician leaders have to say and by what they do. I have three principal windows on clinician leadership, all of which I believe you know about. First, I have been a clinician, staff member, regular observer and occasional organizational consultant in medical education and hospital settings since the Late Bronze Age. Second, I have worked with dozens of physicians and mid-level practitioners in the fellowship programs of the Arizona Center for Integrative Medicine, where I lead modules in spirituality and in health care leadership. Third, I am always drawn to insights from on-the-ground exemplary practice research… particularly, my own research experiences and the Dartmouth Medical School work that I have described.

Let's look at some basic data from these venues… voices of clinicians… and then consider what these data say about health care leadership.

Ten words

In the web-based AzCIM leadership module, I present fellows with some quotations about leadership and invite them to post ten words that speak to what leadership means to them, reflecting on my quotations and their own experiences. The most frequently-cited words are:

- Vision (the clear winner)
- Courage
- Passion

- Integrity
- Clarity (in the sense of direct and forthright communication)
- Presence (and empathy, compassion, caring)
- Inspiring

The best teacher

In workshops about leadership with health care practitioners, I often find it helpful to get the conversation going by inviting participants to describe the best teachers they have had. The qualities of good teachers, usually having to do with inspiring students to do their best, are very much parallel to the qualities of good leaders. A couple of representative responses:

Mr A. was my 11th grade government teacher. Interesting guy… he had come to teaching in his mid-fifties, having worked in publishing for a long time before that. The first words out of his mouth at the beginning of the year were his name (he used his first name rather than "Mister" and I thought that was pretty cool) and "I'm sixty two years old, I've been teaching for seven years and I absolutely love it." He had that infectious enthusiasm all the time… he clearly loved what he was doing and what he was teaching and it rubbed off… it helped me to love it, too.

One of my preceptors in nursing school was a wonderful woman. Nursing school was hard for me… both the work itself and also trying to be a good single mom while I was going through it. She'd take me aside and ask how I was doing and I knew that she genuinely cared. She wasn't just "checking up on a student," but her heart really was in it. I guess the main thing is that I knew that she really believed in me, and that helped me to keep going and made me want to give it everything I could. Over the years, I've tried to be like her with my students.

Definitions of leadership

I also invite AzCIM fellows to define leadership. I am continually impressed with the eloquence and spirit of their responses. Remember, these people are clinicians, primarily mid-career physicians. They are not management experts and, although some of them do some teaching, they are not primarily academics. Some examples:

Leadership is knowing oneself and following one's path with courage, honesty and compassion, while remaining deeply committed to empowering people and community.

The ability to have a vision for the common good, hold it in the mind's eye through all the steps in a day's journey, and have the ability to communicate that vision effectively.

The ability to sit with another long enough that they lean on you when they are relaxed and go to sleep. To have thought through what will come up and to be ready, so when it hits the fan, there is a backup plan, or two, or three.

The ability to build collaboration, inspire people, effectively communicate vision.

Leadership is the accumulation of having a vision, the strength to overcome obstacles, the determination and perseverance to make it through the long haul, the empathy, and compassion to communicate effectively to others your passion, and the willingness to grow with the vision.

Leadership is the ability of a person to inspire others not only by their example, but by their ability to bring out the best qualities of their followers.

Leadership is the ability to motivate and encourage others to reach their individual and collective potential. This can be done on a grand scale with one person influencing people en masse or on a smaller scale by influencing people individually (which through the ripple effect can ultimately become a large number of people).

Behaviors of clinician leaders in exemplary practices

Some observations about leadership from my data on exemplary community health center practices:

There is clearly the expectation in the practice that staff are involved in how the practice works, so that their opinions about how new proposals or policies might affect their jobs are important and valued. (System administrator)

It's so important to be direct with people. The physicians here have nurtured that by being so far from dictatorship, so laissez faire and respectful and empathetic. They create an atmosphere where everybody counts. (Medical records clerk)

When we meet together, Dr. ___ keeps things moving along, but also has the ability to take hold when there is too much tension and start talking calmly and bring everybody down. (Medical assistant)

Every once in a while I get a note from Dr. ___ in a little sealed envelope and it's not about a patient and it's not asking for anything... it's just a positive note saying thanks. She just says something along the lines that patients are really benefiting from my attention and she wants to thank me for being here. She really goes out of her way to express that kind of support. (Nurse)

All the doctors here give me the same warm, personal greeting... it's an expression of "I'm glad to see you," "We're all here together." (Medical assistant)

The doctors are usually rushing around because they have a lot of work to do, but while they're rushing around, they're also acknowledging people and helping everybody if they need something or if somebody needs to talk. (Practice coordinator)

The nurses are wonderful role models. Things can be falling down all around us and their tone of voice and the way that they conduct themselves help to calm things down and defuse tension. They'll get emergency phone calls and defuse things and take the stress out and just deal with the actual facts. (Receptionist)

In the middle of the summer last year, Dr. ___ had a no-show and we all wanted an ice cream bar, so he went out and bought a dozen ice cream bars. I've never heard of that anywhere else. (Medical assistant)

Our providers go above and beyond. All of the outreach they're doing in the community is amazing... Hospice, schools, community health outreach. People see them out in the community giving more of themselves than what they do for a job and that means a lot. (Practice manager)

Dr. ___ is just a wonderful, kind person. I really wanted to come here to work with her. She picks up on how people are doing and will go to someone or take them aside and ask how they are doing and how she can help. It feels good that somebody takes the time to notice how I'm doing and care to ask me about it. (Mid-level practitioner)

He's great as an administrator. He says things with firmness, but always with kindness and respect. You know he's trying to bear everybody's best interests in mind. (LPN)

Dr. ___ really sets the tone. He always says that the patient comes first, no matter how stressed we are. No matter how busy we are, it's the patient that is the most important thing here and they deserve courtesy and professionalism. We all get stressed and harried, but he has a way of reminding us what the priority is and helping us to take a step back and know that it's OK and we'll get through it. (Nurse)

QUALITIES OF SPIRITED HEALTH CARE LEADERSHIP

What do these data say about themes in clinician leadership that make for soulful organizations and good spiritual care? You can cut it a zillion ways, as indeed the management gurus, office-seekers and departed generals organize some of the same basic perspectives on leadership into their own particular frameworks.

Let me describe five themes that I see in these data from health care clinician/leaders, and then I'll invite your reactions.

First, I want to emphasize the idea that leadership need not be limited to formal and defined positions. Leadership arises as anyone takes initiative in some direction that matters to them.

The family physician who championed the birthing room was not in a formal and defined position of leadership. My professional colleague who champions issues of cultural diversity in our organization does not have a formal position or title for doing this; she brings her heart and soul to this because it matters to her and she believes that a continuing focus on honoring cultural diversity will be good for all of us. My administrative support colleague who put up a "brag wall" bulletin board a couple of weeks ago... where people are beginning to post news clippings about their families, poems, and pictures of grandchildren... does not have a job description that says that she should be doing this; it is just an initiative on her part that she believes can help all of us to know one another better and to celebrate the good things in our lives.

Personal wholeness

What leaders *do* is built on a foundation of who leaders *are*. In the data from clinicians, you see reference to "integrity," "her heart was in it," "knowing oneself and following one's path with courage," and "strength... determination... perseverance."

The outward expression of vision and respect cannot arise from a conflicted and chaotic inner life. Quaker theologian Parker Palmer comments,

A leader is a person who has an unusual degree of power to project onto other people his or her shadow, or his or her light. A leader has an unusual degree of power to create the conditions under which other people must live and move and have their being, conditions that can be as illuminating as heaven or as shadowy as hell. A leader must take special responsibility for what is going on inside his or her own self, inside his or her consciousness, lest the act of leadership create more harm than good.[3]

Similarly, from pioneering organizational writers Lee Bolman and Terrence Deal:

Leaders who have lost touch with their own souls, who are confused and uncertain about their core values and beliefs, inevitably lose their way or sound an uncertain trumpet. It is easy to go astray when we forget that the heart of leadership is in the hearts of leaders. We fool ourselves, thinking that sheer bravado or analytical techniques can respond to our deepest concerns. We lose touch with the deepest and most precious of human gifts... soul and spirit. To recapture spirit, we need to relearn how to lead with soul. How to know ourselves and our faith at the deepest level. How to breathe new zest and buoyancy into life. How to reinvigorate the family as a sanctuary where people can grow, develop and find love. How to reinfuse the workplace with vigor and élan. Leading with soul returns us to ancient spiritual basics... reclaiming the enduring human capacity that gives our lives passion and purpose.[4]

Personal wholeness, I believe, is not ultimately about perfection; it is about earnest and heartfelt self-awareness and an ongoing journey of spiritual growth. Heaven help us if we need to be junior Mother Teresas in order to exercise meaningful leadership, but we do need to be accountable to caring about the inner life and how it informs the outer life.

Vision and passion

The clinician data cite "infectious enthusiasm," "vision for the common good," "willingness to grow with the vision," "out in the community... giving of themselves," and "reminding us what the priority is."

Good health care leaders have an intuitive facility with what President Bush the Elder ingloriously referred to as "the vision thing." In practical terms, I think that conversation about vision in leadership refers variously to three component pieces.

First, "vision" often refers to the ability of leaders to **maintain a steady gaze...** and to direct community conversation... **on what**

really matters, and to separate this out from what does not matter as much. The community health center nurse, referring to her physician colleague, notes his reminding the group that "no matter how busy we are, it's the patient that is the most important thing here and they deserve courtesy and professionalism." One can envision this physician in meetings that review budgets, staffing or office practices, anchoring the conversation in the over-arching value that "the patient is the most important thing." Borrowing Koop's phrase, good health care leaders are unfailingly focused on what is "vital and sacred" for the organization and the work that it does.

Second, vision often refers to the ability of leaders to **think creatively.** When someone in a team meeting says, "Let's step back for a minute and re-think the assumptions we are making," or "I may be coming from left field with this, but let me take this conversation in a different direction," you can predict that you are about to hear an item of visionary leadership. In the late 1970s, the initiative of the family physician at the beginning of the chapter was visionary leadership in this sense. His proposal was not to put some new pictures up on the same walls; it was to re-think some of the assumptions about how systems approached labor and delivery.

As we speak of creative thinking, I would remind you of the argument from Chapter 4 about openness to intuition. As we are more spiritually grounded, we become clearer and better able to enter into the flow of intuition, creativity, and wisdom which is all around.

Third, conversation about vision in health care leadership often has a subtext of **passion and enthusiasm.** Not only do you see it; you believe it with all of your heart. How many of us, like the doctor reflecting on his high school government teacher, have been moved by the passion of an attending, preceptor, or mentor?

Passion and inspiration flows in the other direction, too, of course. One of the things that keeps me in the medical education business after lo these many years is the passion and enthusiasm of medical students and young physicians. In the day to day business of health care, it is certainly energizing for me to speak with a young person who is so fresh in their passion about being a healer.

Calming presence

The medical assistant says of the community health center physician, "Dr. ___ keeps things moving along, but also has the ability to take hold when there is too much tension and start talking calmly and bring everybody down." The receptionist speaks of the ability of nurses to "calm things down and defuse tension." The practice coordinator speaks of doctors making time to connect with people in the midst of rushing around.

Clinician leaders in these exemplary practices have the ability to provide a calm and stabilizing presence in the midst of the chaos of everyday medical life. Speaking of refugee boats leaving Vietnam, Thich Nhat Hahn observes that in rough seas, the factor that most consistently helped boats to stay afloat was the presence on board of at least one person who would remain calm and focused. So, too, in health care organizations. When challenging circumstances may prompt a collective wailing and gnashing of teeth, a single person remaining calm and focused can help the team to remain afloat and to pursue more constructive action... as do the physicians and nurses in the exemplary practices.

I might mention that the ability to remain calm and focused in the midst of chaos, for many leaders, represents more than just a personal temperamental quality. It often has to do with assumptions about chaos itself.

The management world has been steadily moving away from a linear, control-based model that is driven by the quest for equilibrium and implemented by top-down decision-making. The newer paradigms, exemplified by thinkers like Peter Senge, emphasize the importance of systems-based ways of looking at organizational life.[5] In these paradigms, the priority is not to remain constant and follow pre-ordained paths, but to cultivate the abilities of work groups to learn from experience and adapt to an inherently changing world. In Senge's view of "learning organizations," for instance, successful performance is associated with employees being able to be open to new ideas and to self-organize around approaches to emerging realities.

With systems models, chaos is no longer the bad guy. Instead, chaos… or perhaps we can be a little less dramatic and say "unforeseen and unpredictable challenges"… provides opportunities for employees and work teams to engage in innovation and self-renewal in ways that help organizations to be more creative and vibrant than they would otherwise be.[6]

The implication of these ideas for health care leadership is that embracing a constantly changing and emerging reality… rather than fearing and resisting it… helps leaders to remain calm and focused.

Integrity

Spirited health care leaders have integrity. The word origin has to do with being "whole," "intact," and "untouched." The word describes personal consistency and uprightness… clarity of values and consistency between words and action.

It has occurred to me that integrity is so important in human experience that it remains undefiled by not having an adjective word form. Have you ever heard the "man (or woman) of integrity" referred to as "integritous" or "integritable?" Integrity is always right there, just what it is.

Our clinician data touch on integrity in references to such qualities as "honesty" and "ability to inspire others… by their example." A community health center nurse cites a particularly striking example of integrity, describing physicians in the practice as being "… out in the community giving more of themselves than what they do for a job," and adding that it "means a lot" that they would do this. Seeing physicians who provide good clinical care extend themselves on personal time on behalf of community causes underscores their commitments to the wholeness and well-being of the populations they serve. It reveals integrity in leadership.

There is a small medical center in southern Maine that prides itself on teamwork, supportive and egalitarian relationships, and on providing patient-centered care.[7] In connection with a project I was doing on health care organizations at the time, I spent part of a day with the medical center CEO. I was impressed. We met in his office, a strikingly unpretentious space with a generic steel desk that had seen better days (I retrieved one just like it from a dumpster at the VA in graduate school... that's another story) and an assortment of Nouveau Thrift Shop furniture and trimmings. He told me that in a challenging economic environment, it was important for him to live with the same financial parameters that he would ask of his employees. Speaking of the commitment to patient-centered care, he described one of his first initiatives when he joined the organization, arranging for himself and his entire board of directors to admit themselves through the ER for an overnight stay in the hospital to experience something of what it was like for patients. We then went on a hospital tour, which was remarkable particularly for his greeting most of his employees personally by name as we went.

The organizational values and the behavior of this health care leader matched up seamlessly. This is integrity.

Encouragement/empowerment

Finally, spirited health care leaders encourage and empower others. Excerpts from our data above include: "empathy," "compassion," "really believed in me," "deeply committed to empowering people," "ability to bring out the best qualities," "ability to motivate and encourage others to reach their individual and collective potential," "their opinions... are valued," and "an atmosphere where everybody counts."

Empowerment means to vest in employees and colleagues the opportunity to make genuine contributions, arising out of their own wisdom and creativity. The operative verbs for empowering leadership are not "tell," "direct," or "manage;" they are "invite," "welcome," and "encourage."

The empowering role of leaders is important for three reasons.

First, ***empowered workers bring their whole selves to work.*** It is said in the business community that managers can control whether or not employees show up and go through their paces, but that employees bring their hearts and souls to work on a volunteer basis.

Part of the success of the exemplary community health centers clearly had to do with the empowering roles of physician, nursing, and administrative leadership.

This is different from other places I've worked. Dr. ___ and [nurse] really want to know what I think about things. Other places, I've gotten the message that my role is to shut up and take blood pressures, but here they actually get after me if I'm too quiet... they expect me to have ideas about how we can be doing things and how we can be working with some of our hard patients. It's great to realize that they really value your opinions... it makes me want to really get out there and work hard with them.

Second, ***empowered work teams are adaptive.*** "Learning organizations," as we considered earlier, are those organizations where front-line work groups have permission and encouragement to be open to new ideas and self-organize responses to new challenges.

Consider the committee meetings you have been involved with over the years. I'd bet you one final pair of Red Sox tickets that the meetings where the participants were largely a listening audience... having only a minimal call for input... were plodding and lifeless. The bet continues... that the meetings where there was a clear agenda, with respect to which everyone's energy and creativity was valued, had a spirit and vitality that was profoundly different.

Third, ***people just have good ideas.*** The pool of good ideas is not exhausted with the contributions of the formal leaders or professional staff. In our organization, some of the best ideas about day-to-day patient flow and procedures have come from staff who are not in defined leadership positions.

As an educational program, moreover, we are always looking to support young physicians in their personal and professional growth, and some of the most perceptive observations about the strengths and vulnerabilities of resident physicians have come from staff.

- *He is outstanding with adolescents… they really trust him.*
- *She works with the hardest and most unappealing patients and gives them real respect.*
- *When she gets out of her routine and unforeseen things come up, she gets curt and inflexible.*
- *I wonder if she is really afraid when she has to say "no" to people who might be abusing narcotics.*

Comments like these, and the conversations that follow, contribute measurably to the educational mission of the organization.

A vital underpinning of the empowering role of leaders is the paradigm of servant leadership.[8] The term comes from Robert Greenleaf, who was an American executive, management consultant, and educator. In a landmark essay in 1970, Greenleaf first described servant leadership, suggesting that effective leaders *serve,* rather than authoritatively *direct,* the people who are responsible to them. This service, according to Greenleaf, has a high regard for people's autonomy, wisdom, personal growth, and well-being. For many years prior to his death in 1990, Greenleaf chaired an institute bearing his name that remains an important source of conferences, seminars, retreats, and educational resources.

STRATEGY 23
Be guided by your own evolving definition of leadership for spiritual care

Be mindful of the importance and form of positive health care leadership. Watch leaders, formal and informal, and reflect on the approaches that empower employees and nurture soulful organizations, and approaches that do not. What works? What does not? What do you respect? What do you not respect?

Write your own definition of spirited leadership, and let that be your guide in one or two initiatives that you can be taking in your organization.

BECOMING A LEADER

How does one become a leader in health care? Are leaders born or made? How can you best contribute to the soul of your organization… or, for that matter, the soul of any social unit you want… your working group, your family, your neighborhood, your community?

Good questions, all. There is, as I have said, no lack of resources about how to become a leader. Rather than presenting you with yet another "12 steps to dynamic leadership success," I'd like to suggest a perspective that I find meaningful and then invite you to engage some self-reflection about the leadership qualities and approaches we have considered.

The perspective comes from Margaret Wheatley, whom you have heard quoted before. Speaking of leadership in organizational life, she says,

The cure for despair is not hope; it is discovering what we want to do about something we care about.

"Discovering what we want to do about something we care about." I love it; simple and elegant. For me, it underscores three important principles about becoming a leader.

First, **all of us are called to leadership.** As we have discussed, we may or may not have formal roles or titles, but any of us has the ability to discover what we want to do about something we care about. The standard for leadership is not any particular office, drawing crowds, or stirring speech; it is taking the initiative to move forward something that matters.

Second, **the energy for leadership arises from "something we care about."** Leadership is driven and energized by our passion of the things that are deeply important to us... we might say, "vital and sacred." The committee to review nursing reorganization. The "bragging" bulletin board. The education of young people in your profession. Creating the kind of team relationships that make you glad to come to work.

Third, *taking initiative with something that matters is not a static point of "deciding;" it is a more fluid process of "discovery."* The family physician at the beginning of the chapter did not jump to the final image of the birthing room on Day One; the final image emerged like sculpture out of the marble from some substantial thought and conversation, and from successive re-visioning and refining the core idea.

Leadership queries

The Religious Society of Friends (Quakers) have a tradition of "queries," occupying much the same space in religious life that creeds and affirmations do in some other religious traditions. Rather than declaring specifically what adherents must believe, the Queries pose questions for self and corporate examination that invite people to reflect on the choices they are making and how their choices fit with the values that are important to them.

The Baltimore Yearly Meeting of the Society of Friends,[9] for instance, invites people to consider:

Do you live in accordance with your spiritual convictions? Do you seek employment consistent with your beliefs and in service to society? Do you practice simplicity in speech, dress and manner of living, avoiding wasteful consumption? Are you watchful that your possessions do not rule you? Do you strive to develop your physical, emotional and mental capacities toward reaching your Divinely given potential? Do you try to direct such emotions as anger and fear in creative ways?

In the spirit of queries in the tradition of Friends, let me invite you to reflect on some of the qualities of leadership that we have explored:

Personal wholeness

- *How do you tend to your own spiritual well-being, so that you may cast light more than darkness upon the people around you?*
- *What does "leading with soul" mean to you? When are the times when you have seen this in yourself? What do you do to bring yourself to a spiritual space where you lead with soul?*

Vision and passion

- *What do you care about?*
- *What do you want to do about what you care about?*
- *How would you hope to see emerging changes in the ways that people receive care in your setting? How would you hope to be caring about the people you work with in 2020?*
- *If time and money were not obstacles, what would you devote your energy and heart towards?*

Calming presence

- *How do you view chaos… or unforeseen and unpredictable challenges? When have there been times when you have been able to embrace change and its creative potential, rather than resisting it?*
- *When have you been able to maintain a calm spirit and focused presence in the midst of chaos? How do you do this?*

Integrity

- *In what ways do you inspire others by your example?*
- *How does you behavior align with your personal and organizational values? What might you do to further strengthen this alignment?*

Exercise Empowering Leadership

Encouragement/empowerment

- *When have there been times when you have been able to help bring out the best that is in other people?*
- *What do you do to affirm and encourage the wisdom, creativity and initiative of people you work with?*
- *In what ways do you see yourself as a servant of the people whom you lead?*

And I'd add a final query, returning to Richard McKnight's reflection that begins this chapter:

- *How might you grow in your encouragement of people "through meaning, love and hope?"*

STRATEGY 24
Pick one or two points of growth for yourself as a leader with soul.

Reflect on these queries and choose one or two areas could be potential points of growth for you as a leader. Focus some time and your attention and heart on these areas... being mindful, creating some space for self-reflection, perhaps journaling, perhaps speaking with people you care about. Allow these aspects of your leadership to root more deeply and find widening expression in your life.

SUMMARY

- Positive health care leadership is essential to providing good spiritual care.
  - o Exercising good leadership is good for the soul.
  - o Good leadership helps staff to be engaged in their work and supportive of one another.
  - o Good leadership ultimately benefits patients, because good leadership forms good organizational culture, and soulful organizations provide good spiritual care.

- Qualities of spirited health care leadership include:
  - o Personal wholeness; what leaders do is built upon a foundation of who leaders are.
  - o Vision and passion: good leaders maintain steady and passionate focus on what really matters and think creatively about pursuing it.
  - o Calming presence: good leaders maintain a calm and focused presence, sustained by the assumption that chaos is not the bad guy… but that chaos often presents opportunities for employees and work teams to engage in innovation and self-renewal.
  - o Integrity: spirited leaders inspire others by example, and give expression to personal and organizational values in their behavior.
  - o Encouragement/empowerment: good leaders bring out the best in other people, encouraging their wisdom, creativity, and initiative.
- Becoming a leader may be thought of as "discovering what we want to do about what we care about."
  - o Regardless of position, we are all called to leadership in the sense of moving forward things that matter.
  - o Leadership is driven and energized by our passion for the things that are deeply important to us.
  - o Taking initiative with something that matters is not a static point of "deciding;" it is a more fluid process of "discovery."

REFERENCES

1. McKnight R. Spirituality in the workplace. In: Adams J, ed. *Transforming Work: A Collection of Organizational Transformation Readings.* Alexandria, VA: Miles River Press; 1984:139-153.

2. Schein E. *Organizational Culture and Leadership, 2nd ed.* San Francisco, CA: Jossey-Bass; 1997.

3. Palmer P. Leading from within. In: Conger J, ed. *Spirit at Work: Dis-*

covering the Spirituality in Leadership. San Francisco: Jossey-Bass; 1994.

4. Bolman LG, Deal TE. *Leading with Soul: An Uncommon Journey of Spirit.* San Francisco: Jossey-Bass; 2001.

5. Senge P. *The Fifth Discipline: The Art and Practice of the Learning Organization.* New York: Doubleday; 1990.

6. Pascale R, Milleman M, Gioja L. *Surfing the Edge of Chaos: The Laws of Nature and the New Laws of Business.* New York: Three Rivers Press; 2001.

7. Mann P. Lobster rolls and room service. *Down East.* 1998 (November): 70-73, 88-79.

8. Greenleaf R, Vaill P, Spears. *The Power of Servant Leadership.* San Francisco, CA: Berrett-Koehler; 1998.

9. *Faith and Practice of Baltimore Yearly Meeting.* Baltimore, MD: Baltimore Yearly Meeting; 1988.

AFTERWORD

At the end of a workshop a couple of years ago, a participant came up to me and asked how I would summarize what we had considered together about spirituality and health care in one sentence. Great question; I have learned that some of the best questions and conversations in my sessions with groups take place after the program is over and most people are making their way out the door.

The challenge, of course... as you have by now correctly concluded... is that I am not the sound byte guy. I am somehow constitutionally better able to expand an idea into five pages than to contract it into one.

Nonetheless, the question was intriguing. It reminded me of cereal boxtop contests growing up: Write "Why I love Coco Puffs" in fifteen words or less and win a chance at a genuine Dick Tracy two-way wristwatch radio.

My response to the workshop participant was,

Be curious about what it is like to be somebody else and keep an open heart.

I'm not sure that this is the definitive sentence, and I might very well say something else if you asked me tomorrow... but it does touch on ideas that have always been deeply meaningful for me. Such as holding the people who come into our lives in an attitude of wonder about what it is like to have their life experience and what it might mean for them to live out what is "vital and sacred" for them. And holding people... ourselves included... in a place of honor, openness to spirit, and love in our own hearts.

I also don't presume that this needs to be the definitive sentence for you. I have thought of this book as a conversation that affirms your experience and your wisdom, along with suggesting some ideas that arise out of the experiences that I have had.

In that spirit, I'd invite you to answer this woman's question for yourself. How would you put into words the boxtop summary of what "Positive Spirituality in Health Care" means to you? What might you particularly bear in mind for yourself, your patients, and your health care organization moving forward? What do you take pride in, that you have always taken pride in, that brings goodness into your world? What might be one or two new ideas you could focus on until you visit these questions again?

Your picking up this book certainly makes you a kindred spirit, and you have my best wishes and blessings.

Fred

Waterville, Maine
June, 2009

APPENDIX I

A Dozen of Fred's Favorite
Spirituality and Health Websites

As we accelerate our movement in to the digital age, there is a stunning proliferation of Internet resources about everything, spirituality and health included. I'm sure you have some favorite websites. Here are a dozen of mine, in no particular order.

Spirituality & Health

http://www.spirituality-health.com/spirit/

Website of the long-running Spirituality & Health magazine. Articles by prominent authors on soulful living… "body," "soul," and "earth." Full-text content of current issues available a few weeks after publication, along with searchable full-text archives of past issues. Forums, eCourses, newsletter, self tests about spiritual well-being, gratitude, forgiveness and other subjects.

This I Believe

http://thisibelieve.org/

Inspired by 1950s radio program hosted by Edward R. Murrow, *This I Believe* is a nonprofit organization that solicits and distributes short essays about people's core values that guide their daily living. Famous people, regular folk, many with extraordinarily compelling stories to tell. Published in book and CD format, the essays are most widely available as a weekly feature and podcast on NPR. Website has a "browse essays by theme" feature… creativity, kindness, hope, parenthood, etc.

Portraits of Grief

http://www.nytimes.com/pages/national/portraits/

Faced with the decision about how to recognize the 9/11 victims, the New York Times decided to run non-traditional obituaries that would forgo the usual recitation of formal accomplishments in favor of celebrating something of the spirit and character of the people who perished. A remarkable collection of anecdotes and images… a generous spirit, a prankster, a voice of calm, a great barbeque artist. Searchable by name (including my colleague Frederick Rimmele III, MD) but best browsed. Breaks your heart and lifts your soul.

The George Washington Institute for Spirituality and Health
http://www.gwish.org/
Founded in 2001 by Christina Puchalski, MD, GWISH is involved with medical education, research, and interdisciplinary initiatives in spiritual care. Partners with the John Templeton Foundation on a number of projects, notably grants to medical education programs for spirituality curriculum development and a beginning Spirituality and Health Online Education and Resource Center (SOERCE). New multimedia guide to spiritual assessment, featuring the FICA spiritual history tool.

The Fetzer Institute
http://www.fetzer.org/
Michigan-based, internationally-prominent nonprofit encouraging the power of love and forgiveness in individuals and systems. Great audio and video collections… Desmond Tutu, Parker Palmer, and His Holiness the Dalai Lama, among many others. Significant print resources, including monographs on spirituality in community and public life, and on multidimensional instruments for measuring religiousness and spirituality in health research.

The Forgiveness Web
http://www.forgivenessweb.com/
Comprehensive compilation of forgiveness resources… articles, books, videos, links. Good sub-sections; grief, self-forgiveness, sexual abuse, The Holocaust, among others. Extraordinarily touching "Apology Room," where people anonymously post messages seeking forgiveness and affirming life change.

Gratefulness.org
www.gratefulness.org
Brother David Stiendl-Rast, OSB, is certainly one of the leading
contemporary writers on the subject of gratitude. Website has articles, an inventory of gratitude practices, some lovely visual images,
and not-to-be-missed "virtual candle-lighting" exercise.

Health Progress
http://www.chausa.org/Pub/MainNav/News/HP/
Health Progress is a bi-monthly journal published by the Catholic
Health Association of the United States. A publication venue for a
large number of practical articles about spirituality and health care,
leadership, and organizational culture. Searchable subject index for
each issue, full-text available back to 1992.

Institute for Research on Unlimited Love
http://www.unlimitedloveinstitute.org/
Website coordinated by Stephen Post, PhD, Professor, Department
of Bioethics, Case School of Medicine at Case Western Reserve.
Research summaries, articles, links about altruism, compassion and
service.

Institute of Noetic Sciences
www.noetic.org
IONS is a nonprofit organization that "conducts and sponsors
leading-edge research into the potentials and powers of consciousness—including perceptions, beliefs, attention, intention, and intuition. The institute explores phenomena that do not necessarily fit
conventional scientific models, while maintaining a commitment
to scientific rigor." The name "noetic" refers to "inner knowing"
or "intuitive consciousness." Research, electronic and print publications, events, retreat center. Searchable keyword index to full-text
IONS publications from websites and journals.

Appreciative Inquiry

http://appreciativeinquiry.cwru.edu

Exciting movement in the world of systems and organizational development, focusing not on remediating system problems but on finding and drawing out the best in people and organizations, the "systematic discovery of what gives 'life' to a living system when it is most alive, most effective, and most constructively capable." Site has research, extensive bibliography with links to text, assessment and training tools and links specifically to Appreciative Inquiry in Medicine.

Værdsættende samtale

http://www.vaerdsaettende-samtale.dk/

Værdsættende Samtale er en særlig udviklingsform, der gør en organisation i stand til selv at forbedre sit arbejdsmiljø og virkeevne. Denne portal sigter mod at skabe forbindelser mellem mennesker der interesserer sig for Værdsættende samtale. (Mainly, I am checking to see if you are paying attention, but if you are interested in Appreciative Inquiry and happen to speak Danish, this site is for you!)

Positive Psychology

http://www.positivepsychology.org

Portal for background, exercises and resources about Positive Psychology and character strengths and virtues. Standardized self-tests for optimism, signature strengths, compassionate love, and meaning in life, among others.

APPENDIX II

A Fiddler's Dozen of Fred's Favorite Books on Spirituality and Health Care

New books on spirituality and health care have been sprouting like seedlings underneath my maple trees. Here are a dozen and a half good resources, thirteen of which have been published since 2003. (You will see that 2006 was a banner year.) Written by a wonderful range of folks… physicians, counselors, spiritual care specialists, nurses, educators… they offer a rich variety of perspectives and narratives about working with spiritual resources and issues.

Carson VB, Koenig HG. *Spiritual Caregiving: Healthcare as a Ministry.* 2004. West Conshohocken, PA: Templeton Foundation Press. Carson is a PhD nurse educator and Koenig is a physician with a background in geriatric medicine and psychiatry who is director and founder of the *Center for the Study of Religion/Spirituality and Health* at Duke. Oriented to caregivers, with "goal of providing healthcare professionals and caregivers the inspiration and practical tools to re-claim their sense of purpose." Reflections on dealing professionally with intense distress and on spiritual self-care, with personal narratives from a variety of voices in health care.

Haynes WF, Kelley GB. *Is There a God in Health Care?: Toward a New Spirituality of Medicine.* 2006. Binghamton, NY: Haworth Pastoral Press. A cardiologist and a theologian present cases and reflect on "how personal faith can enhance the immune system, how a spiritual outlook can help bear the burden of suffering and grief, and how forbearance and forgiveness are crucial in maintaining a healthy attitude toward life." Sections on prayer, faith and illness, lessons from the healing ministry of Jesus, forgiveness and reconciliation in the healing process.

Hodge DR. *Spiritual Assessment: Handbook for Helping Professionals.* 2003. Botsford, CT: National Association of Christians in Social Work. Varieties of assessment methodologies… spiritual history-taking, spiritual lifemaps, spiritual ecomaps, spiritual genograms, spiritual "ecograms"… with examples of applications.

King DE. *Faith, Spirituality, and Medicine: Towards the Making of the Healing Practitioner.* 2000. Binghamton, NY: Haworth Pastoral Press. Exploration of the relationship between patient health and traditional religious beliefs and practices. Background about spirituality and health, assessing spirituality, ethics, chaplaincy, short section on integrating spirituality in practice. Author is a family physician.

Kliewer S, Saultz J. *Healthcare and Spirituality.* 2006. Radcliffe. Kliewer is a pastoral caregiver who has been active in the spirituality interest group of the Society of Teachers of Family Medicine. Saultz is a family physician and educator. Designed as "an introductory textbook." Background on spirituality and health, cultures and beliefs of different religious traditions, spiritual assessment and spiritual intervention ("creating trust, creating awareness, stimulating change, facilitating change"). Many case examples and good questions for reflection.

Koenig HG. *Spirituality in Patient Care: Why, How, When, and What (2nd Ed.).* 2007. West Conshohocken, PA: Templeton Foundation Press. Good descriptions of opportune circumstances in health care in which to address patients' spirituality and approaches with which to do this. Excellent summary of literature on spiritual assessment and collection of resources, circa 2002. Oriented more to "religion" than to "spirituality" per se. Helpful chapter on "When religion is harmful" and handling religious conflicts.

McSherry W. *Making Sense of Spirituality in Nursing and Health Care Practice: An Interactive Approach.* 2006, London and Philadelphia: Jessica Kingsley Publishers. Perspectives on spirituality (spiritual needs, spiritual distress, spiritual well-being), relevance of spirituality to health care, approaches and barriers to spirituality in health care, skills needed, and implications for education.

Miller, WR (Ed.) *Integrating Spirituality into Treatment.* 1999. Washington, DC: American Psychological Association. Excellent scholarly overview with ample practical illustrations and recommendations. Great chapters on mindfulness, prayer, spiritual surrender, acceptance and forgiveness, hope, and serenity.

O'Hanlon B. *Pathways to Spirituality: Connection, Wholeness, and Possibility for Therapist and Client.* 2006. New York: Norton. Spirituality as "connection," "compassion," and "contribution." Practical, touched by O'Hanlon's ever-present sense of humor, and intersects with his substantial work in the solution-focused therapy movement.

Orchard H (Ed.). *Spirituality in Health Care Contexts.* 2001. London and Philadelphia: Jessica Kingsley Publishers. Chapters by researchers and clinicians from the UK about spirituality in institutions, professional issues of chaplains, and perspectives of different faith traditions.

Puchalski, CM. **A Time for Listening and Caring: Spirituality and the Care of the Chronically Ill and Dying.** 2006. New York: Oxford University Press. Director of the George Washington Institute of Spirituality and Health, Dr. Puchalski has been a prolific author and advocate for the incorporation of spirituality in health care. Sections on spirituality in relationships, spiritual and religious healing traditions, and practical approaches, particularly in the settings of serious illness and end of life care. Nice emphasis on patients' stories.

Shea, J. *Spirituality & Health Care: Reaching toward a Holistic Future.* 2000. Park Ridge, IL: The Park Ridge Center. Reflections on spirituality with respect to patients, caregivers, chaplains, organizations, and medical ethics. Nice section on "welcoming spiritualities" and hospitality of health care organizations.

Sorajjakool S, Lamberton H (Eds). *Spirituality, Health, and Wholeness: An Introductory Guide for Health Care Professionals.* 2004. Binghamton, NY: Haworth. Sorajjakool is professor of religion, psychology, and counseling at Loma Linda University. Chapters on wholeness and mind/body/spirit connections, trauma, illness and meaning, and spirituality in working with "difficult patients," among others.

Sorajjakool S. *When Sickness Heals: The Place of Religious Belief in Healthcare.* 2006. West Conshohocken, PA: Templeton Foundation Press. Perspective that health crises can lead to renewed sense of meaning in life and a "reconfiguration of belief systems in order to accommodate chronic or terminal illness." Cases, cross-cultural illustrations.

Sulmasy, DP. *The Rebirth of the Clinic: An Introduction to Spirituality in Health Care.* 2006. Washington, DC: Georgetown University Press. Author is a physician and Franciscan Friar. Explores the meaning of health, illness, and healing, with particular reference to end of life care. Nice section on "Taking physicians' oaths seriously."

White BF, Mac Dougall JA. *Clinician's Guide to Spirituality.* 2001. New York: McGraw-Hill. Published by McGraw-Hill in collaboration with the Hazelden Foundation (the addictions treatment organization). Written by a physician and a chaplain, presents a universal model of spirituality that is independent of religion, and shows how the clinician can apply the model to help in the management of chronic illness. Twelve principles of spirituality applied to health: honesty, hope, faith, courage, integrity, willingness, humility, compassion, justice, perseverance, spiritual awareness, service.

White G. *Talking About Spirituality in Health Care Practice: A Resource for The Multi-Professional Health Care Team.* 2006. London and Philadelphia: Jessica Kingsley Publishers. Written by a dietician in the UK who has worked in palliative care and convened groups of colleagues to explore together how spirituality informs their practice. Considers the nature of spirituality, how this is approached in multidisciplinary teams and ways of "developing opportunities to talk about spirituality."

Young C, Coopsen C. *Spirituality, Health and Healing.* 2006. Sudbury, MA: Jones and Bartlett Publishers. Authors are founders of an organization that provides continuing education to nurses. Book is intended as a resource in spiritual care for providers of health care and pastoral care. Content includes exploring the spiritual dimension of individuals, the various aspects of spiritual care, spiritual dimensions in particular types of care, and spiritual considerations of special populations.

About the Author

Frederic C. Craigie, Jr., PhD graduated magna cum laude from Dartmouth College and subsequently received MS and PhD degrees in Clinical Psychology from the University of Utah. He served two years of internships in the Veterans Administration system in Maine and Utah.

Since 1978, he has been a faculty member at the Maine-Dartmouth Family Medicine Residency in Augusta, Maine. He also holds appointments as Associate Professor of Community and Family Medicine at Dartmouth Medical School and Visiting Associate Professor at the Arizona Center for Integrative Medicine (AzCIM) at the University of Arizona College of Medicine.

Dr. Craigie has a longstanding interest in spirituality and heath care. Over the last 25 years, he has written and presented extensively about the healing and life-giving roles of spirituality in patient care, in the experience of health care providers, and in the life and culture of health care organizations.

With the Arizona Center for Integrative Medicine, Dr. Craigie has taught about spirituality and health care for the Fellowship and Integrative Medicine in Residency programs since 2001. He received a John Templeton Spirituality and Medicine Award for Primary Care Residency Training Programs (in conjunction with

George Washington University Medical Center, Institute for Spirituality and Health) in 2002. He is also the founder of a pastoral care program at the Residency's affiliated hospital, the organizer of an annual Maine symposium on spirituality and health care since 1987, and has served for many years as associate editor of a professional journal devoted to Christian faith and mental health.

In his personal life, Fred finds joy in his relationships with his wife, Beth, and grown children, Heather (and Matt), Matthew, and Tom. In addition, he pursues his own spirituality by playing fiddle and Appalachian dulcimer, running up and down the court playing basketball three or four times a week, doing carpentry, and resolutely following the subtleties and wonders of major league baseball. He has called Maine "home" since the mid-seventies.

INDEX